Plant Medicines for Clinical Trial

Plant Medicines for Clinical Trial

Special Issue Editor

James David Adams

MDPI • Basel • Beijing • Wuhan • Barcelona • Belgrade

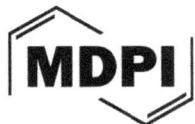

MDPI

Special Issue Editor
James David Adams
University of Southern California
USA

Editorial Office
MDPI
St. Alban-Anlage 66
Basel, Switzerland

This is a reprint of articles from the Special Issue published online in the open access journal *Medicines* (ISSN 2305-6320) from 2016 to 2018 (available at: http://www.mdpi.com/journal/medicines/special_issues/clinical_trial)

For citation purposes, cite each article independently as indicated on the article page online and as indicated below:

LastName, A.A.; LastName, B.B.; LastName, C.C. Article Title. *Journal Name* **Year**, *Article Number*, Page Range.

ISBN 978-3-03897-023-1 (Pbk)
ISBN 978-3-03897-024-8 (PDF)

Cover image courtesy of James David Adams.

Contents

About the Special Issue Editor

James David Adams, PhD, Associate Professor examines the chemistry and clinical uses of California medicinal plants. He was trained for 14 years by a Chumash Indian Healer. Dr. Adams practices traditional California healing and writes about the pharmacological basis for the use of plant medicines. He has written several papers that teach one how to cure chronic pain with plant medicines. If these medicines can be tested in clinical trials and used in modern medicine, many thousands of lives will be saved from opioid and nonsteroidal anti-inflammatory drug toxicity.

Preface to "Plant Medicines for Clinical Trial"

Plant medicines are natural medicines that humans have always used. Many people continue to use plant medicines today including teas, coffee, chocolate, ginger, tobacco, marijuana, and other medicines. Traditional medicine is based on plant medicines and is the primary form of medicine for many people throughout the world. The current volume discusses traditional medicines and presents various plant medicines that could be tested in clinical trials. Modern medicine continues to use many drugs that are derived from plants. The current work has much to teach modern medicine about the treatment of several diseases. Traditional healers have used plant medicines to treat psychiatric and other conditions that modern medicine struggles with. Safety issues are always a concern with plant medicines, especially allergies to plant medicines. Clinical trials must be conducted with plant medicines to help bring these traditional treatments into use by modern medicine.

Modern medicine, especially cancer medicine, seeks drugs from plant medicines. Single purified agents from plants are tested in clinical trials and may become accepted medicines in the clinic. The modern attitude is that medicines are magic bullets that find single targets in the body to treat disease. Modern medicine hopes that the magic bullet approach will minimize drug toxicity. However, every drug is toxic, depending on the dose. We human beings have used crude plant medicines for our entire existence. Our bodies have adapted to and evolved with crude plant medicines that have kept us alive.

We do not purify single nutrients from our foods. We eat crude fruits and vegetables. Our bodies benefit from many constituents in our food. Purifying the protein out of a fruit eliminates the fiber that helps with blood sugar and cholesterol. We forget that the body is the most powerful medicine we have. Treating the body of a cancer patient as if it were a flask of cancer cells is dangerous. It may be better to follow a short course of therapy with a period of recuperation that allows that body to heal itself and eliminate the cancer.

Prevention should be the basis of modern medicine. We should learn from Traditional Healers about how to live in balance and let our bodies heal themselves. We can prevent heart disease, type 2 diabetes, osteoarthritis, and cancer.

James David Adams
Special Issue Editor

medicines

MDPI

Editorial

Does the World Need Plant Medicines?

James David Adams

School of Pharmacy, University of Southern California, Los Angeles, CA 90089-9121, USA; jadams@usc.edu

Received: 19 April 2018; Accepted: 19 April 2018; Published: 23 April 2018

Our species has always used plants as medicines, during our 200,000 year existence. This is made obvious by the plant medicines found in mummy burials, around the world, dating back thousands of years. Human beings evolved using plant medicines to stay alive. This has resulted in a genetic selection in which those who were healed by plant medicines and survived were able to pass on their genes. Modern humans must continue to use plant medicines.

When a Traditional Healer is asked how her people learned how to use a specific plant medicine, the answer is usually that God taught them. Each of us has a spiritual sense that can be used to seek answers [1]. Finding a new plant medicine involves fasting, praying, and spending as much as four days with the plant that will become a new medicine [2]. Traditional Healers are still the major or only source of healthcare for many regions of the world. The loss of Traditional Healers in some areas has resulted in major changes in healthcare, sometimes to the detriment of the people [3,4]. Since Traditional Healers may be religious leaders also, they provide moral direction for the community. The displacement of traditional religious beliefs has been detrimental in some regions.

The most powerful medicine each person has is the human body. The body heals itself. When the body is in balance, it can heal itself of many conditions, in other words, it can prevent many diseases [5,6]. Patients should be taught what balance is and how to maintain balance, including staying thin and strong.

Drugs are not magic bullets that cure diseases. They help the body heal itself. Even antibiotics and anticancer drugs are of no use when the immune and defense systems are not functioning well. In many clinical trials, the placebo works as well as the drug because of the body's ability to heal itself [7].

Clinical trials are useful to demonstrate what a plant medicine can be used to treat and to demonstrate safety. Useful information can be derived from placebo controlled clinical trials, from clinical trials that compare a new medicine to an old medicine and from other clinical trial designs. Many different clinical trial designs are appropriate. The double blind, randomized, placebo controlled clinical trial should not be used as the gold standard of clinical trial design [7]. Many other designs are just as valid and may be less risky to patients, such as patients who are put on the placebo.

Clinical trials are frequently abused. Drugs are shown to help with one disease symptom and are approved for use, even though they are very toxic. Many of the oral medicines used to treat pain are dangerous drugs that kill many patients. Oral opioids kill about 67,000 people in the USA every year. Oral nonsteroidal anti-inflammatory drugs have been estimated to kill at least 50,000 USA patients every year from ulcers, heart attacks, and strokes [8,9]. The most dangerous way to treat pain is with oral or injected pain medications. Some of the drugs approved for type 2 diabetes cause heart disease. Some of the drugs approved for heart disease cause type 2 diabetes. Just because a drug is useful for one symptom, does not mean the drug should be used.

Drugs are frequently used as if they were the only possible treatment for a disease. Patients seem to have become convinced that drugs can take care of any disease. Prevention is the best treatment for many chronic diseases that plague the modern world. Type 2 diabetes, heart disease, and osteoarthritis are caused by excess visceral fat, obesity [10,11]. Visceral fat secretes toxic lipids and akipokines that cause these diseases. Toxic adipokines also potentiate the formation of cancer in the body [10].

As modern man has become more sedentary and obese, these diseases have increased greatly, much to the benefit of the pharmaceutical industry. A better option is to live in balance and prevent diseases.

In the midst of our crisis of drug over use and abuse, patients must find alternative choices for healthcare. Prevention should always be the healthcare of choice. When medicines are needed, many plant medicines continue to be available in most of the world. In the United States, medicines are tightly regulated by the Food and Drug Administration. Due to this strict regulation, few indigenous American plant medicines are readily available. Patients must find Traditional Healers who still know how to make Native American plant medicines [2]. Plant medicines made from European plants are much more available in the United States.

In the current publication, Edenta, Okoduwa, and Okpe teach about the use of plant medicines in Nigeria [12]. *Musa acuminata* is a species of banana that originally comes from Southeast Asia and has been cultivated for over 8000 years. It was probably introduced into Nigeria long ago. Traditional Healers in Nigeria use *M. acuminata* peels in the treatment of their patients. There are several cultivars of *M. acuminata*, each with different pharmacology and toxicology. The work of Edenta and coworkers demonstrates that some plant medicines may not be safe for human use.

Kinda et al. discuss the use of plant medicines to treat neuropsychiatric conditions by Traditional Healers in Burkina Faso [13]. Neuropsychiatric conditions existed during ancient times and were a burden for the community. In traditional villages, each member of the village has a job that is critical to the survival of the village. If a neuropsychiatric condition prevented a village member from being productive, the Traditional Healer had to find a way to help. In Burkina Faso, Traditional Healers use 66 different plant species to make medicines for neuropsychiatric conditions. Modern medicine relies on the use of dopamine 2 receptor antagonists to treat psychosis. These drugs cause extrapyramidal side effects in 50% of patients, weight gain in most patients, and potentially irreversible tardive dyskinesia in 68% of patients treated for 25 years. Even though dopamine 2 receptor antagonists are useful in neuropsychiatric conditions, their toxicity is a concern. Modern medicine may be wise to learn from the Traditional Healers of Burkina Faso.

Tchuenmogne et al. describe their work to find biologically-active compounds from *Terminalia mantaly*, the Madagascar almond [14]. They describe several compounds that are interesting antifungal agents. Pathak, Upreti, and Dikshit provide evidence of antifungal compounds from a lichen, *Usnea orientalis* [15]. The treatment of fungal infections has become very important and difficult due to the huge increase in type 2 diabetes in the world. Diabetics are very susceptible to fungal infections.

Balogun et al. examine an endangered medicinal plant, *Oncoba spinosa*. This small tree grows in many areas of Africa [16]. The fruit is used in Traditional Healing in Nigeria. Although several reports have examined the Phytochemistry of the plant, Balogun and coworkers found a compound not previously seen in the leaves. The compound, flacourtin, is also found in an Indian plant that is used in Traditional Healing.

Al-Tamimi, Rastall, and Abu-Reidah report on the antioxidant and toxic properties of nine essential oils [17]. In order to produce an essential oil, a large amount of plant material is heated, such as in a steam bath, until the volatile compounds from the plant distill. Essential oils have been used in European Traditional Healing. Some essential oils are very toxic, even to the skin. El-Tamimi and coworkers found that ginger, chamomile, and African rue essential oils were of interest. They also found that some essential oils are not pharmacologically potent and suggest that storage and preparation conditions may be important with these products.

Ouedraogo and Kiendregeogo discuss the antibiotic potency of *Anogeissus leiocarpus*, African birch [18]. The plant is used by Traditional Healers in wound healing. Methanol extracts of the plant were examined against bacterial strains. This work shows the importance of wound healing in traditional villages. There are probably several alternative treatments that modern medicine should consider for the treatment of difficult wounds, such as diabetic skin ulcers.

Santos et al. present evidence of cytotoxic and antimicrobial compounds in an essential oil from *Lippia alba*, bushy mattgrass, which comes from the Caribbean, Central and South America [19].

They found 39 compounds, of which many are monoterpenes. Some monoterpenes from bushy mattgrass may be useful against fungal infections.

Khurm et al. provide evidence of the safety of *Heliotropium strigosum*, called Kharsan, Gorakh pam, and Bhangra in Pakistan [20]. The plant is used in Traditional healing for respiratory and GI problems. Plant preparations have low toxicity against several bacteria and fungi. The medicine is known to contain compounds that relax inflamed lung tissue.

Work from my laboratory, by Wang et al., provides controversial evidence for the use of a plant medicine in the treatment of Alzheimer's disease [21]. In ancient times, some older people suffered from what is now called Alzheimer's disease. Chumash Healers found that the berries of *Heteromeles arbutifolia*, toyon, a California plant, helped slow down the progression of the disease. White people labeled the plant poisonous, due to their racist beliefs that plants used by Indians must be poisonous. The plant has not been carefully examined until now. My group found several interesting compounds in the plant and demonstrated the safety of the berries in several patients. All of the clinical trials of new Alzheimer's disease drugs have failed [22]. Perhaps this plant medicine should be examined in clinical trials.

Olorunnisola, Fadahunsi, and Adegbola teach us about Traditional Healing with *Sphenocentrum jollyanum*, aduro kokoo. The plant is used as a medicine in several West African countries [23]. Alkaloids, saponins, flavonoids, and other compounds are found in the plant. Traditional Healers have found several uses for the plant in treating their patients, including high blood pressure. Black Americans are resistant to several antihypertensive drugs. It may be wise to use this plant in resistant patients.

Rodriguez Villanueva, Esteban, and Rodriguez Villanueva discuss the use of *Marrubium vulgare*, horehound in type 2 diabetes [24]. The authors find that clinical trials performed with the plant were flawed. They suggest finding better clinical trial methods in order to accurately assess the value of the plant. This is a constant problem in plant medicine clinical trials. In the USA, the Food and Drug Administration and the National Center for Complementary and Integrative Health insist on using hydro-alcoholic extracts of American plants or similar preparations in clinical trials, even though Traditional Healers have never used these preparations. The purpose of these clinical trials, therefore, is to disprove the efficacy of the plant medicines. This is a vivid reminder of the anti-Indian racism that permeates these federal agencies.

Teng et al. provide a case report of a woman who had a successful pregnancy after being treated with Chinese herbal medicines. In vitro fertilization had failed in the woman [25]. This case reinforces the power of herbal medicines.

The purpose of the current writing is to educate the healthcare community about the importance of plant medicines. Plant medicines can be safe and efficacious even when modern drugs fail. Plant medicines should be used in the traditional preparations and by the traditional routes. One of the advantages of plant medicines is that they contain several active compounds that all add to therapy. They may even potentiate or synergize the effects of other compounds in the medicine. The author of the current writing encourage the modern use of plant medicines after performing realistic clinical trials.

Conflicts of Interest: The author declare no conflict of interest.

References

1. Adams, J.; Garcia, C. The spiritual sense, prayer and traditional American Indian healing. *TANG Int. J. Genuine Tradit. Med.* **2012**, *2*, 1–6. [CrossRef]
2. Garcia, C.; Adams, J. *Healing with Medicinal Plants of the West—Cultural and Scientific Basis for Their Use*, 3rd ed.; Abedus Press: La Crescenta, CA, USA, 2016.
3. Adams, J. What can traditional healing do for modern medicine? *TANG Hum. Med.* **2014**, *4*, 1–6. [CrossRef]
4. Adams, J. Is something wrong with modern medicine? *Indian Country Today* **2012**, *1*, 11.
5. Adams, J. *The Balanced Diet for You and the Planet*; Abedus Press: La Crescenta, CA, USA, 2014.
6. Adams, J. Preventive Medicine and the Traditional Concept of Living in Balance. *World J. Pharmacol.* **2013**, *2*, 73–77. [CrossRef]

7. Adams, J. Design flaws in randomized, placebo controlled, double blind clinical trials. *World J. Pharmacol.* **2011**, *1*, 4–9. [CrossRef]

8. Adams, J. Chronic pain—Can it be cured? *J. Pharm. Drug Dev.* **2017**, *4*, 105–109.

9. Adams, J.; Haworth, I.; Coricello, A.; Perri, F.; Nguyen, C.; Aiello, F.; Williams, T.; Lien, E. The treatment of pain with topical sesquiterpenes. In *Frontiers in Natural Product Chemistry*; Atta-Ur-Rahman, Ed.; Bentham Science Publishers: Sharjah, UAE, 2017; Volume 3, pp. 176–195. ISBN 978-1-68108-535-7.

10. Adams, J.; Parker, K. (Eds.) *Extracellular and Intracellular Signaling*; Royal Society of Chemistry: London, UK, 2011. [CrossRef]

11. Peplow, P.; Adams, J.; Young, T. (Eds.) *Cardiovascular and Metabolic Disease Scientific Discoveries and New Therapies*; Royal Society of Chemistry: London, UK, 2015.

12. Edenta, C.; Okoduwa, S.I.R.; Okpe, O. Effects of Aqueous Extract of Three Cultivars of Banana (*Musa acuminata*) Fruit Peel on Kidney and Liver Function Indices in Wistar Rats. *Medicines* **2017**, *4*, 77. [CrossRef] [PubMed]

13. Kinda, P.T.; Zerbo, P.; Prosper, T. Guenné, S.; Compaoré, M.; Ciobica, A.; Kiendrebeogo, M. Medicinal Plants Used for Neuropsychiatric Disorders Treatment in the Hauts Bassins Region of Burkina Faso. *Medicines* **2017**, *4*, 32. [CrossRef] [PubMed]

14. Tchuenmogne, M.A.T.; Kammalac, T.N.; Gohlke, S.; Kouipou, R.M.T.; Aslan, A.; Kuzu, M.; Comakli, V.; Demirdag, R.; Ngouela, S.A.; Tsamo, E.; et al. Compounds from *Terminalia mantaly* L. (Combretaceae) Stem Bark Exhibit Potent Inhibition against Some Pathogenic Yeasts and Enzymes of Metabolic Significance. *Medicines* **2017**, *4*, 6. [CrossRef] [PubMed]

15. Pathak, A.; Upreti, D.K.; Dikshit, A. Antidermatophytic Activity of the Fruticose Lichen *Usnea orientalis*. *Medicines* **2016**, *3*, 24. [CrossRef] [PubMed]

16. Balogun, O.S.; Ajayi, O.S.; Lawal, O.S. Isolation and Cytotoxic Investigation of Flacourtin from Oncoba spinosa. *Medicines* **2016**, *3*, 31. [CrossRef] [PubMed]

17. Al-Tamimi, M.A.; Rastall, B.; Abu-Reidah, I.M. Chemical Composition, Cytotoxic, Apoptotic and Antioxidant Activities of Main Commercial Essential Oils in Palestine: A Comparative Study. *Medicines* **2016**, *3*, 27. [CrossRef] [PubMed]

18. Ouedraogo, V.; Kiendrebeogo, M. Methanol Extract from Anogeissus leiocarpus (DC) Guill. et Perr. (Combretaceae) Stem Bark Quenches the Quorum Sensing of Pseudomonas aeruginosa PAO1. *Medicines* **2016**, *3*, 26. [CrossRef] [PubMed]

19. Santos, N.O.D.; Pascon, R.C.; Vallim, M.A.; Figueiredo, C.R.; Soares, M.G.; Lago, J.H.G.; Sartorelli, P. Cytotoxic and Antimicrobial Constituents from the Essential Oil of Lippia alba (Verbenaceae). *Medicines* **2016**, *3*, 22. [CrossRef] [PubMed]

20. Khurm, M.; Chaudhry, B.A.; Uzair, M.; Janbaz, K.H. Antimicrobial, Cytotoxic, Phytotoxic and Antioxidant Potential of *Heliotropium strigosum* Willd. *Medicines* **2016**, *3*, 20. [CrossRef] [PubMed]

21. Wang, X.; Dubois, R.; Young, C.; Lien, E.J.; Adams, J.D. Heteromeles Arbutifolia, a Traditional Treatment for Alzheimer's Disease, Phytochemistry and Safety. *Medicines* **2016**, *3*, 17. [CrossRef] [PubMed]

22. Lien, E.; Adams, J.; Lien, L.; Law, M. Alternative approaches to the search for Alzheimer's disease treatments. *J. Multidiscip. Sci. J.* **2018**, *1*, 2. [CrossRef]

23. Olorunnisola, O.S.; Fadahunsi, O.S.; Adegbola, P. A Review on Ethno-Medicinal and Pharmacological Activities of Sphenocentrum jollyanum Pierre. *Medicines* **2017**, *4*, 50. [CrossRef] [PubMed]

24. Villanueva, J.R.; Esteban, J.M.; Villanueva, L.R. A Reassessment of the Marrubium Vulgare L. Herb's Potential Role in Diabetes Mellitus Type 2: First Results Guide the Investigation toward New Horizons. *Medicines* **2017**, *4*, 57. [CrossRef] [PubMed]

25. Teng, B.; Peng, J.; Ong, M.; Qu, X. Successful Pregnancy after Treatment with Chinese Herbal Medicine in a 43-Year-Old Woman with Diminished Ovarian Reserve and Multiple Uterus Fibrosis: A Case Report. *Medicines* **2017**, *4*, 7. [CrossRef] [PubMed]

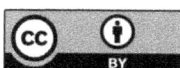

medicines

MDPI

Review

A Review on Ethno-Medicinal and Pharmacological Activities of *Sphenocentrum jollyanum* Pierre

Olubukola Sinbad Olorunnisola, Olumide Samuel Fadahunsi * and Peter Adegbola

Department of Biochemistry, Faculty of Basic Medical Sciences, Ladoke Akintola University of Technology, Ogbomoso, PMB 4000, Oyo State, Nigeria; osolorunnisola@lautech.edu.ng (O.S.O.); useablevesselofgod@gmail.com (P.A.)
* Correspondence: fadahunsiolumide5@gmail.com; Tel.: +23-470-3384-3022

Academic Editor: James D. Adams
Received: 10 June 2017; Accepted: 28 June 2017; Published: 3 July 2017

Abstract: *Sphenocentrum jollyanum* Pierre is a member of a diverse family of plants known as Menispermaceae. They are famous for a plethora of important biological functions. *S. jollyanum* is a shrub native to the tropical forest zones of West Africa and thrives in deep shade. It is widely cultivated in Cameroun, Sierra Leone, Nigeria, Ghana, and Côte d'Ivoire. *S. jollyanum* is employed in folk medicine as a cure for wounds, fever, coughs, high blood pressure, breast tumor, constipation, and as an aphrodisiac. Phytochemical investigations revealed that the plant is a rich source of secondary metabolites such as annin, alkaloids, saponins, and flavonoids. Pharmacological activities include anti-diabetic, anti-inflammatory, anti-bacterial, anti-viral, anti-malarial, angiogenic, and anxiogenic. Thus, this present review summarizes the phytochemical and nutritional constituents and important biological studies on various crude extracts, fractions, and isolated principles of all morphological organs of *S. jollyanum*.

Keywords: ethno-medicinal uses; pharmacological activities; phytochemical profile; *Sphenocentrum jollyanum* Pierre

1. Introduction

Globally, the employment of medicinal plants as a substitute for orthodox drugs in the management of various diseases has been increasing due to the unavailability of modern health facilities, relative availability of medicinal herbs, poverty, and recent revelations that they possess active compounds that may be responsible for different biological and pharmacological actions [1]. According to Newman and Cragg [2], natural materials are the source of about two -third of all drugs developed in the past three decades. According to a World Health Organization (WHO) report, it is estimated that close to 80% of the people living in the third world nations of the world depend on traditional and complementary medicines for their basic health care [3]. Thus, this review is aimed at elucidating the traditional and biological importance of *Sphenocentrum jollyanum*.

S. jollyanum Pierre is a member of the plant family Menispermaceae (Table 1). These are diverse group of plants which are popular for important biological activities. *S. jollyanum* is a shrub native to the tropical forest zones of West Africa and is widely distributed in Sierra Leone, Nigeria, Ghana, Ivory Coast, and Cameroun [4]. It is extensively employed in folkloric medicine in the management of various ailments. *S. jollyanum* is commonly known locally as *"Aduro kokoo"* (red medicine), *"Okramankote"* (dog's penis), and *"Krakoo"* among the Akan and Asante tribes of Ghana. In South-Western Nigeria, the plant is traditionally known as Akerejupon or Ajo, Oban abe in Republic of Benin, and Ouse-abe in Côte d'Ivoire [5].

2. Plant Description

Sphenocentrum jollyanum (Figure 1) is a perennial under growth of dense forest, which thrives in deep shade, from sea-level up to 400 m altitude. It is mostly found in regions withmean annual rainfall of 1800 mm or more, mean minimum temperature of 20 °C, and mean maximum of 29 °C. It grows to an average height of about 1.5 m, with few scanty branches. *S. jollyanum* leaves are wedge-shaped, about 5–12 cm wide, smooth onboth sides, and can grow up to about 20 cm long with a small-arrowed apex [6,7]. The fruit (Figure 2) occurs as clusters, ovoid-ellipsoid, with a single large oval-shaped seed. It is fleshy, edible, and bright yellow or orange when ripe [8,9]. The roots are visibly bright yellow and are characterized by a sour acidic taste that causes things eaten thereafter to taste sweet [8].

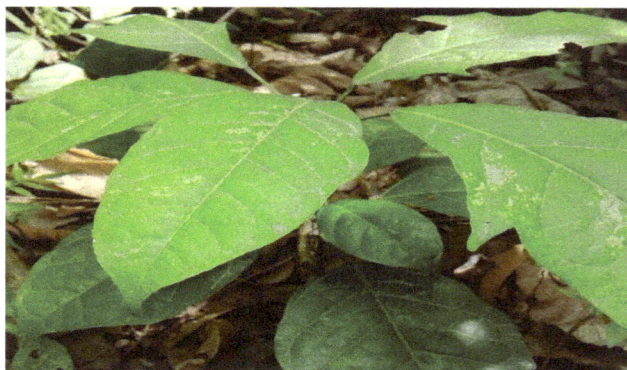

Figure 1. *Sphenocentrum jollyanum* in its natural habitat.

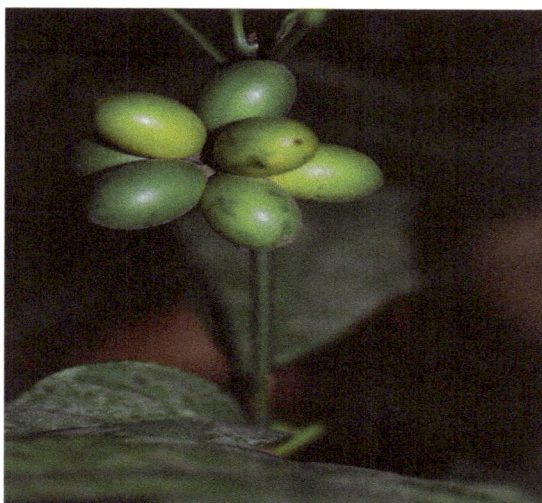

Figure 2. *Sphenocentrum jollyanum* fruits.

Table 1. Taxonomical classification of *Sphenocentrum jollyanum* [5].

Kingdom	Plantae
Division	Magnoliophyta (Cronquist)
Subdivision	Magnoliophytina (Frohne and Jensen)
Class	Ranunculopsida (Brongn)
Subclass	Ranunculidae (Takht)
Suborder	Ranunculanae (Takht)
Order	Menispermales (Bromhead)
Family	Menispermaceae (Juss.)
Genus	Sphenocentrum (Pierre)
Species	Jollyanum

3. Ethno-Medicinal Uses

Different parts of *S. jollyanum* are traditionally employed in folkloric medicine. In Ghana, the root of the plant is widely used by the men as an aphrodisiac. It is steeped in alcohol for few days to allow extraction of some constituents, which is thereafter drank as bitters to strengthen penile erection, and this effect is known to be long-lasting [10,11].

It has been documented in several literature studies that the root is employed for its effectiveness in stimulating the central nervous system (CNS), the management of mental and inflammatory disorders, pain and depression [12]. The dried, powdered root is used in combination with some anti-malarial plant as panacea for fever and muscular pains. Aerial parts of the plant (leafy twigs and fruits) are vastly employed in the treatment of chronic wounds, feverish conditions, and coughs when combined with *Piper guineense* (West African pepper) and lime juice [8,9].

In Nigeria, the roots are chewed in traditional medicine to relieve constipation, promote appetite, and increase digestion. All morphological organs of *S. jollyanum* are important ingredients in the management of sickle cell disease (SCD) [8]. Traditional healers in Ghana and Côte d'Ivoire have also reported the roots to possess medicinal properties against high blood pressure, breast tumor, irregular menstrual cycle, and diabetes mellitus [7,13–16]. Furthermore, the powdered roots are eaten in combination with *Aframomum melegueta* (alligator pepper) seeds, salt, and *Elaeis guineensis* (African oil palm) in the management of abdominal discomfort [17]. The charred fruits are used in the treatment of fibroids and as edible anti-fatigue snack [9,18]. It is also reported that the leaves decoctions are used in expelling intestinal parasites and to stop spitting of blood [15].

4. Phytochemical and Proximate Analysis

The majority of the reported biological and pharmacological activity of *S. jollyanum* extracts (Table 2) has been attributed to their bioactive principles and constituent phytochemicals. A detailed phytochemical analysis of the ethanol root extract of *S. jollyanum* revealed that it contains compounds such as terpenoids and flavonoids, while alkaloids are reported to be the most dominant chemical constituents [19]. Phytochemical investigation by Nia et al. [4] revealed the presence of tannins, saponins, terpenes, and alkaloids in the different fractions of methanol extracts of the stem bark. The chloroform fraction was found to be the most active of all fractions, and it tested positive to the test of flavonoids and alkaloids. In the submission of Aboabaand Ekundayo [20], detailed analysis of the essential oil of *S. jollyanum* root using gas chromatography-mass spectrometry analysis (GC-MS) revealed a total of 19 compounds (α-pinene, α-ylangene, guaia-6,9-diene-4α-ol, globulol, guaiene-11-ol, α-eudesmol, isocaryophyllene, aromadendrene, selina-4(15),6-dien E-β-isocaryophyllene, γ-terpinene, γ-humulene, epi-zonarene, δ-amorphene, 1,8-cineol,camphene, B-pinene, p-cymene, d3-carene, Figure 3) consisting of monoterpenoids (33.5%) and sesquiterpenoids (56.3%), while (10.2%) of the total oil constituents remain unidentified. Phytochemistry of the seed extracts by Ibironke et al. [21] revealed the bio-availability of flavonoids, alkaloids, and saponins, while phylobatannin and free anthraquinone were not present. Proximate analysis of the seed extract showed the crude fat, moisture, crude protein, carbohydrate, ash, and fiber contents to be 9.65%, 16.70% 48.09%, 16.79%, 3.26%, and 5.51%, respectively, while the energy value was 1460 kcal/100 kg. This suggests that the fruits are an important source of nutrients and energy [21]. Interestingly, the flame photometric and atomic absorption spectrophotometric (AAS) analysis of the mineral element composition of the seeds showed an appreciable amount of macro and micro elements that are required for the growth in humans and animals [21]. Minerals such as calcium (8.92 mg/L), magnesium (0.44 mg/L), potassium (4.26 mg/L), iron (0.22 mg/L), manganese (0.19 mg/L), zinc (1.38 mg/L), and sodium (4.70 mg/L) were present in appreciable quantity. This indicates the importance of the plant in building strong bones, the production of energy, and carrying out some metabolic reactions in the body [21]. Previous scholarly articles documented the isolation of three furanoditerpenes (columbin, isocolumbine, and fibeucin) (Figure 4) and alkaloids (protoberberine) from the fruit [22].

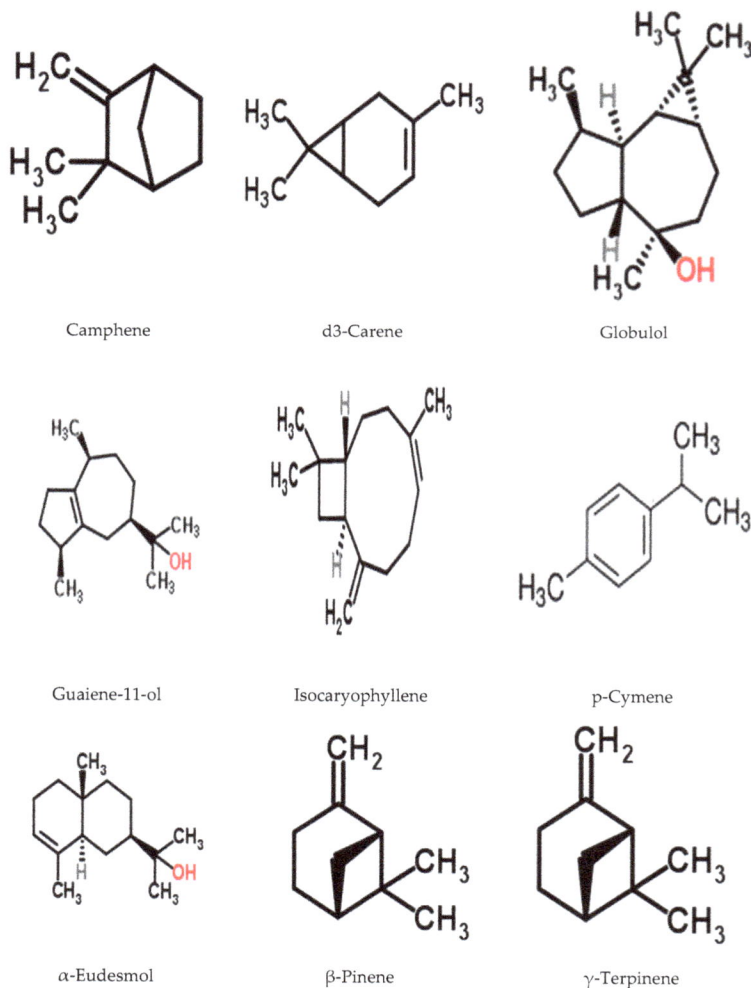

Camphene	d3-Carene	Globulol

Guaiene-11-ol	Isocaryophyllene	p-Cymene

α-Eudesmol	β-Pinene	γ-Terpinene

Figure 3. Some identified compounds from the root oil of *S. jollyanum*.

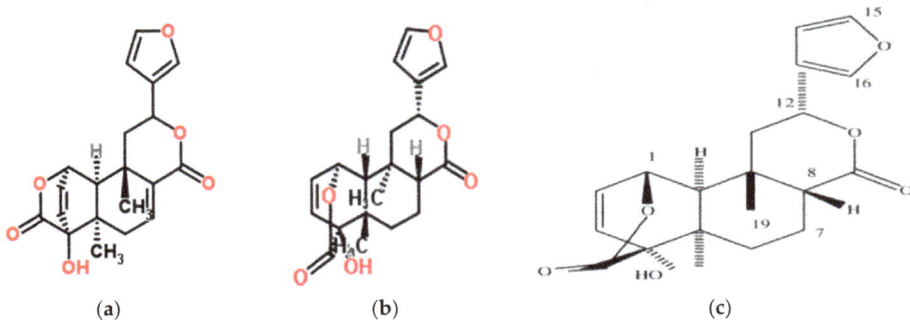

Figure 4. Isolated compounds from fruits of *S. jollyanum*. Structure of isolated fibleucin (**a**) and isocolumbin (**b**) [22], Structure of isolated columbine (**c**) [22].

Table 2. Summary of pharmacological activities *of S. jollyanum*.

Pharmacological Activities	Part Used	Extracts	References
Angiogenic	Stem bark,	Methanol, Chloroform	[4]
Anti-Oxidant	Stem bark, Root, Leaf	Methanol, Hexane, Chloroform, Ethanol, Butanol, Aqueous	[4,23,24]
Anti-Bacteria	Root	Essential oil, Ethanol	[20,25]
Haematological	Leaf , Root	Methanol	[22,23,26]
Anti-Inflammatory	Fruit, Root,	Methanol, Ethanol, Aqueous	[22,27,28]
Anti-Diabetic	Root, Stem, Fruit, Leaf	Aqueous, Ethanol, Methanol	[29–32]
Hypolipidemic	Root	Ethanol	[32]
Hepatoprotective,Toxicological	Stem bark, Leaf, Root,	Methanol, Ethanol, Essential oil	[23,26,33]
Anti-Malaria	Leaf, Root	Methanol	[24,34]
Weight Loss Prevention	Leaf , Root, Seed	Ethanol, Essential oil	[24,26,33,35]
Anti-Allergy	Fruit	Ethanol	[36]
Anti-viral	Stem, Root, Leaf	Hexane, Methanol	[37,38]
Anti-depressant	Root	Ethanol	[39]
Anxiogenic	Root	Ethanol	[40,41]
Analgesic, Antipyretic	Leaf	Methanol	[42]
Sexual, Reproductive	Root	Ethanol, Methanol	[43,44]

5. Pharmacological and Biological Activities

5.1. Anti-Diabetic Activity

Investigation of the different extracts of morphological organs of *S. jollyanum* indicated its blood glucose lowering potential. The effect of petroleum ether seed extract on oral glucose tolerant test (OGTT) and alloxan-induced diabetic rabbits revealed that 1 g/kg of the extract administered 30 min before glucose load considerably reduced blood glycemic level by 20% relative to the untreated group. The study also reported the anti-hyperglycemic activity of the extract on alloxan-induced diabetic rabbits [29]. In another study, a 9-day treatment regimen revealed that the extract caused a significant ($p < 0.05$) dose-dependent decrease in the plasma glucose level from the 3rd to the 9th day. The three-dosage group showed a peak percentage decrease of 12.3%, 29.2%, and 32.7%, which compared favorably with glinbenclamide at 51.9%. Furthermore, the aqueous root extract demonstrated a dose-dependent reduction in blood glycemic level of alloxan-induced diabetic rabbits [30]. Ethanol extracts of *S. jollyanum* leaf at concentrations of 50, 100, 200 mg/kg significantly

($p < 0.05$) lowered the blood glycemic index of alloxan-induced diabetic rabbits in a dose-dependent manner, with plasma glucose level of 200.2 mg/100 mL (42.8%) at 200 mg/kg [31]. Alese et al. [32] reported that the methanol root extract demonstrated hypoglycemic effects on streptozotocin-induced diabetic Wistar rats. Oral dosage of 200 mg/kg extracts for 2 weeks caused a significant decrease in blood glucose to 6.62 mmol/L relatively to the uncontrolled group with blood glucose level of 16.3 mmol/L. The results of these studies validate the traditional claim of the blood glucose lowering activity of the plant, and thus may serve as a potential source of potent anti-diabetic compounds.

5.2. Antioxidant Activity

Studies on superoxide radical and hydrogen peroxide scavenging ability of the methanolic stem extract revealed a dose-dependent anti-oxidant activity with IC_{50} value of 13.11 µg/mL and 30.04 µg/mL when compared to ascorbic acid 15.34 µg/mL and 35.44 µg/mL respectively [23]. In a separate study, Olorunnisola and Afolayan[24] reported that the plant significantly ($p < 0.05$) ameliorated the oxidative stress related with *P. berghei* infection in mice, which was evident in the reduced levels of total protein and liver MDA (malondialdehyde). In addition, there was increased activity of serum and liver catalase (CAT), superoxide dismutase (SOD) and glutathione (GSH) levels. Alternatively, Nia et al. [4] point to the anti-oxidant activity of extracts of all morphological organs on 2,2-diphenyl-1-picrylhydrazyl hydrate (DPPH). The stem bark was observed to be the most active with IC_{50} of 1.80 µg/mL, when compared with ascorbic acid 0.80 µg/mL. The leaf had the weakest activity, IC_{50} of 4.35 µg/mL, while IC_{50} of the root bark was 3.50 µg/mL. Fractions of the stem bark were screened, and the chloroform fraction exhibited the most potent activity with an IC_{50} of 1.54 µg/mL. The findings emanating from these studies indicate the potential of *S. jollyanum* as an anti-oxidant (Table 2), and thus could be explored in the development of new pharmaceuticals.

5.3. Anti-Inflammatory

Studies on the in vivo anti-inflammatory activity of *S. jollyanum* crude extracts and isolated compounds were investigated in healthy adult rats inoculated with carrageenan [22]. It was reported that the methanol fruit extract at a concentration of 200 mg/kg showed the stronger inhibition (79.58%) of oedema formation on hind paws, while root extract demonstrated a 53.75% inhibition. The same study also revealed that three furanoditerpenes (namely columbin, isocolumbine, and fibleucin) isolated from the methanolic fruit extract demonstrated considerable anti-inflammatory potentials. Columbin and flavonoids-rich fraction at 200 mg/kg exhibited 67.08% and 76.25% anti-inflammatory activities that were in a comparable range with acetylsalicylic acid. Olorunnisola et al. [27,28] evaluated the in vitro inflammatory potential and possible modes of action of crude extracts and secondary metabolites of *S. jollyanum* organs. The results also provided some vindication for the traditional usage of *S. jollyanum* in managing inflammatory-related diseases in the West African sub-region.

5.4. Anti-Allergy Activities

The anti-allergic study was performed on milk-induced leukocytosis and oesinophilia in mice. The ethanolic fruit extracts demonstrated a considerable dose-dependent decrease in the absolute eosinophil and lymphocyte counts. The results suggested the anti-allergy property of the fruit extract, and the mode of activity may involve multiple mechanisms due to phytochemical interactions [36].

5.5. Anti-Malarial Activities

Anti-malarial studies on the leaf and root extracts of *S. jollyanum* were reported by Olorunnisola in [24,34] respectively. The in vivo anti-plasmodial activity of methanol extracts was evaluated using chloroquine-resistant *Plasmodium berghei* NK67 strain-inoculated *S*wiss albino mice. The leaf and root extracts demonstrated statistically significant concentration-dependent activities of (74.4%) and (54.1%), respectively. However, the standard drug arthemether-lumefartrin had a better antimalaria activity (81.4%). Further research is necessary to identify and characterize the active components and determine the possible mode of activity.

5.6. Anti-Bacterial Activities

Aboaba and Ekundayo [20] studied the essential oil composition of the root extract of *S. jollyanum* against *Bacillus subtilis*, *Salmonellatyphi*, *Staphylococcus aureus*, *Bacillus cereus*, *Proteus mirabilis*, and *Pseudomonas aeruginosa*. It was observed that the essential oil was effective against *Bacillus subtilis* and *Pseudomonas aeruginosa* strains with inhibition zones of 10 mm and 9.0 mm, respectively, at 1000 µg/mL. In a separate study, Koleosho et al. [25] showed the plant extract to be a potent inhibitor of *S. typhi*. The moderate antimicrobial activity displayed supports the traditional use of the root as a laxative which aids proper bowel movements and digestion.

5.7. Anti-Viral Activities

Moody et al. [37,38] revealed that the methanol extracts of the different morphological parts were assessed for their antiviral activities on polio virus Types 1, 2, and 3. It was observed from the study that the leaf and root extracts were active against polio virus Type 2. Additionally, hexane and methanol extracts were investigated and reported for their mosaic virus inhibitory potentials in cowpea.

5.8. Haematological Activities

Methanol root and leaf extracts of *S. jollyanum* were investigated for possible hematopoietic activity in Wistar mice infected with chloroquine-resistant *Plasmodium berghei* NK67. Methanol extracts of leaf and root were administered orally for 7 days. The study revealed that there was a significant increase in the pack cell volume (PCV), mean corpuscular volume (MCV), mean corpuscular hemoglobin concentration (MCHC), and hemoglobin (Hb). There was also an observable elevation in red and white blood cell levels, with the exception of monocytes and neutrophils. The study is suggestive of the ability of the extract to stimulate hematopoietic stem cells [22,23,26].

5.9. Effect on Weight

The effect of leaf and root extracts on weight change was investigated in malaria and diabetic rat. It was observed that there was a significant ($p < 0.05$) increase in weight gain in Wistar mice treated with the extracts. Comparative analysis suggested that the extracts significantly prevented loss of weight in a concentration-dependent pattern in the extract-administered group when compared to the negative control [24,26,33,35]. Consequently, the physical status of the extract-treated animals was improved. This may be related to the ameliorative effect of the extracts to prevent the acute fluid loss, fat catabolism, and protein catabolism which are evident in weight loss.

5.10. Hepatoprotective and Toxicological Studies

Scientific examination of the hepatoprotective potential of stem bark extract revealed that the extract significantly ameliorated/prevented liver damage in carbon tetrachloride (CCl_4)-induced rats. The study showed that the extract considerably ($p < 0.05$) reversed the elevated aspartate aminotransferase (AST), alkaline phosphatase (ALP), alanine amino transferase (ALT), and total bilirubin, and decreased the level of total serum protein in a concentration-dependent pattern [23]. In the submission of Mbaka et al. [26,33], no mortality or morbidity was recorded in the 120-days administration of ethanol leaf extract during the toxicity studies. Detailed assessment also indicated that there was no obvious inflammation of the internal organs. In addition, there were no appreciable increases in serum AST and ALT in the extract-administered animals. This observation denotes that the extract poses no damaging effect on the liver. The result of the histological study on the liver tissue morphology confirmed that no toxic effects of the extract were visible. Furthermore, minimum cytotoxic dose (MCD50) of the methanol leaf extract was also investigated on Hep-2 (Human epithelia cell line) and it was found to range within 3.9×10^{-3} mg/mL [37]. The Ames microbial mutagenicity test of the root ethanol extract showed no statistically observable increase in the number of revertant colonies in the four strains of *S. typhimurium* TA_{97}, TA_{98}, TA_{100}, and TA_{102} at any concentration. This indicates that *S. jollyanum* has no ability to cause mutation in relation to the in vitro assay [19]. According to Aboaba and Ekundayo [20], the toxicity of the essential oil of *S. jollyanum* to brine shrimp lethality test showed a lethal concentration LC_{50} of 84.87 ppm. Therefore, the observed safety level of the plant extracts vindicates its age-long ethno-pharmacological usage.

5.11. Hypolipidemic Activity

Effect of the ethanol root extract on serum lipid profile was investigated on streptozotocin-induced diabetic albino rats. It was noticed that there was no observable difference in total cholesterol (TC) amount of the extract- and glinbenclamide-administered animals. Additionally, there was a significant ($p < 0.02$) difference in antiartherogenic index (AAI) and high-density lipoprotein level in extract-treated group (0.77 ± 0.02 mmol/L) when compared to untreated infected group (0.85 ± 0.02 mmol/L) [32].

5.12. Antidepressant Activity

The anti-depressant effect of the ethanol extract of the root was evaluated on mice using forced swimming and tail suspension examination. The plant extract (100–1000 mg/kg) increased the duration of mobility in both models in a concentration-dependent manner. However, it was observed that the standard drugs imipramine and fluoxetine were 20–50 times more potent than the extracts. This implied that the antidepressant activity of the extract might be as a result of its modifying activity on monoamine transport and metabolism [39].

5.13. Anxiogenic Activity

Anxiogenic activity was carried out by administration of 100–1000 mg/kg of the ethanol extract. The animals exhibited anxiety-like effects dose-dependently in a similar way to those induced by caffeine (10–100 mg/kg), and this was in contrast to the anxiolytic effect of diazepam (0.1–1 mg/kg) [40,41]. The result validates the conventional use of the plant for its stimulatory effect on the central nervous system and as mood enhancer.

5.14. Anti-Angiogenic Activity

Angiogenesis has been reported as a fundamental process in the transition of benign tumors to malignant ones, and therefore Nia et al. [4] evaluated the anti-angiogenic activities of the methanol extract of morphological organs using in vivo chick chorioallantoic membrane (CAM) angiogenesis assay. It was revealed that the stem bark had the most potent activity, with an IC_{50} value of 1.00 μg/mL. In addition, the chloroform fraction of the stem bark exhibited the strongest inhibitory IC_{50} (1.54 μg/mL) activity against the formation of new endothelial cells [4], thus validating the ethno-botanical usage of *S. jollyanum* as an important anti-tumor agent.

5.15. Antipyretic and Analgesic Activities

Muko et al. [42] disclosed that the petroleum ether and methanol extracts of *S. jollyanum* leaves possess significant in vitro analgesic and antipyretic activities.

5.16. Reproductive and Sexual Activity

Investigation on the potential of the plant extracts to affect sexual activities and hormonal levels in laboratory animals was carried out by Owiredu et al. [43]. It was observed that there was an increased urge by the male animals to mount on the female for the first time, increased duration of ejaculation, and shortened refractory period. Furthermore, a decrease in post-ejaculatory, climbing and intromission latency was observed in the extract-treated animals. These are relevant perceptions of sexual performance and satisfaction. In addition, testosterone level was increased by four-fold and about there was a one-third increment in follicle stimulating hormone (FSH) activity. However, there was a contradictory report by Raji et al. [44] that pointed to a considerable reduction in the total sperm count, fertilization ability of the sperm cells, movement and swimming (asthenozoospermia) abilities. There was also a considerable increase in superoxide dismutase activity in relation to the testes and degeneration of seminiferous tubules. However, it was suggested that *S. jollyanum* could produce deleterious effects on reproductive ability, which can be measured as a function of poor sperm quantity (epididymal sperm count), quality (sperm movement, viability, structure), and gradual impairment, loss of function of the tissues and cells of the testes.

6. Conclusions

The importance of *S. jollyanum* in the traditional medicinal system of Africa cannot be over-emphasized. The medicinal value of the plant is owed to it richness in alkaloids, tannins, saponins, flavonoids, and essential oils. These bioactive principles have been reported to be responsible for the various pharmacological efficacies reported in this review. Hence, all morphological organs of the plant stand an important chance as a major source of potent therapeutic compounds useful in the management of several human diseases.

Author Contributions: O.S.O. conceived the idea and outlined the content, O.S.F. and P.A. searched the internet and wrote the manuscript. All authors read and approved the final manuscript for submission.

Conflicts of Interest: Authors declare there is no conflict of interest.

References

1. Tiwari, A.K.; Mehta, R. Medicinal plants used by traditional healers in Jashpur district of Chhattisgarh India. *Life Sci. Leafl.* **2013**, *1*, 31–41.
2. Newman, D.J.; Cragg, G.M. Natural products as sources of new drugs over the 30 years from 1981 to 2010. *J. Nat. Prod.* **2012**, *75*, 311–335. [CrossRef] [PubMed]
3. Farnsworth, N.R.; Akerele, O.; Bingel, A. Medicinal plants in therapy. *Bull. World Health Organ.* **1985**, *63*, 965–981.
4. Nia, R.; Paper, D.H.; Essien, E.E. Evaluation of the anti-oxidant and anti-angiogenic effects of *Sphenocentrum jollyanum* Pierre. *Afr. J. Biomed. Res.* **2004**, *7*, 129–132.
5. Amidu, N. An Evaluation of the Central and Sexual Behavioral Effects and Toxicity of the Root Extract of *Sphenocentrum jollyanum* Pierre (Menispermaceae). Ph.D. Thesis, Department of Molecular Medicine, Kwame Nkrumah University of Science & Technology, Kumasi, Ghana, 2008.
6. Dalziel, J.M. *The Useful Plants of West Tropical Africa*; Crown Agents: London, UK, 1985.
7. Iwu, M.M. *Handbook of African Medicinal Plants*; CRC Press: Boca Raton, FL, USA, 1993; p. 239.
8. Abbiw, D.K. *Useful Plants of Ghana*; Intermediate Technology Publications and Royal Botanic Gardens: Kew, UK, 1990.
9. Neuwinger, H.D. *African Ethno Botany: Poisons and Drugs*; Chapman and Hall: London, UK, 1996.
10. Irvine, F.R. *Woody Plants of Ghana: With Special Reference to the Uses*; Oxford University Press: London, UK, 1961.
11. Burkill, H.M. *Volume 1: The Useful Plants of West Tropical Africa*; Royal Botanical Gardens: Kew, UK, 1985.
12. Oke, J.M.; Hamburger, M.O. Screening of some Nigeria medicinal plant Antioxidant Acitivity Using 22-Diphenyl-picryl-hydrazyl radical. *Afr. J. Biomed. Res.* **2002**, *5*, 77–79.
13. Odugbemi, T. *Medicinal Plants by Species Names: Outlines and Pictures of Medicinal Plants from Nigeria*; Lagos University Press: Ojo, Lagos State, Nigeria, 2006.
14. Oliver-Bever, B. *Medicinal Plants in Tropical West Africa*; Cambridge University Press: Cambridge, UK, 1986.
15. Kayode, J.; Ige, O.E.; Adetogo, T.A.; Igbakin, A.P. Conservation and Bio derversity in Ondo State, Nigeria. Survey of plant barks used in native pharmaceutical extraction in Akoko region. *EthnoBot. Leafl.* **2009**, *13*, 665–667.

16. Fasola, T.R.; Egunyomi, A. Bark extraction and uses of some medicinal plants. *Niger. J. Biotechnol.* **2002**, *15*, 23–36.

17. Ghana Herbal Pharmacopoeia. *Ghana Herbal Pharmacopoeia*; Advent Press: Accra, Ghana, 1992.

18. Egunyomi, A.; Fasola, T.R.; Oladunjoye, O. Charring Medicinal Plants: A Traditional Method of Preparing Phytomedicines in Southwestern Nigeria. *EthnoBot. J.* **2005**, *3*, 261–265. [CrossRef]

19. Amidu, N.; Woode, E.; Owiredu, K.B.; William, A.; George-Boateng, A.K.; Opoku-Okrah, C. An Evaluation of Toxicity and Mutagenicity of *Sphenocentrum jollyanum*. *Int. J. Pharm.* **2008**, *4*, 67–77.

20. Aboaba, S.A.; Ekundayo, O. Constituents, antibacterial activities and toxicological assay of essential oils of *Artocarpus communis* Forst (Moraceae) and *Sphenocentrum jollyanum* (Menispermaceae). *Int. J. Biol. Chem. Sci.* **2010**, *4*, 1455–1461. [CrossRef]

21. Ibironke, A.A.; Olusola, O.O. Phytochemical analysis and mineral element composition of ten medicinal plant seeds from South-west Nigeria. *N. Y. Sci. J.* **2013**, *6*, 2–28.

22. Moody, J.O.; Robert, V.A.; Connolly, J.D.; Houghton, P.J. Anti-inflammatory activities of the methanol extracts and an isolated furanoditerpene constituent of *Sphenocentrum jollyanum* Pierre (Menispermaceae). *J. Ethnopharmacol.* **2006**, *104*, 87–91. [CrossRef] [PubMed]

23. Olorunnisola, O.S.; Akintola, A.A.; Afolayan, A.J. Hepatoprotective and antioxidant effect of *Sphenocentrum jollyanum* (Menispermaceae) stem bark extract against CCl4-induced oxidative stress in rats. *Afr. J. Pharm. Pharmacol.* **2011**, *5*, 1241–1246. [CrossRef]

24. Olorunnisola, O.S.; Afolayan, A.J. In Vivo antioxidant and biochemical evaluation of *Sphenocentrum jollyanum* leaf extract in *P. berghei* infected mice. *Pak. J. Pharm. Sci.* **2013**, *26*, 445–450. [PubMed]

25. Koleosho, A.T.; Jose, A.R.; Oyibo, P.G.; Roland-Ayodele, M.A.; Uloko, M.E. Antimicrobial Activity of *Sphenocentrum jollyanum* and *Mangifera indica*Linn On *Salmonella Typhi*. *Pak. J. Pharm. Sci.* **2013**, *5*, 50–54.

26. Mbaka, G.O.; Adeyemi, O.O.; Oremosu, A.A. Acute and sub-chronic toxicity studies of the ethanol extract of the leaves of *Sphenocentrum jollyanum* (Menispermaceae). *Agric. Biol. J. N. Am.* **2010**, *1*, 265–272. [CrossRef]

27. Olorunnisola, O.S.; Fadahunsi, O.; Adetutu, A.; Olasunkanmi, A. Evaluation of Membrane Stabilizing, Proteinase and Lipoxygenase Inhibitory Activities of Ethanol Extract of Root and Stem of *Sphenocentrum jollyanum* Pierre. *J. Adv. Biol. Biotechnol.* **2017**, *13*, 1–8.

28. Olorunnisola, O.S.; Fadahunsi, O.S.; Owoade, O.A. In Vitro anti-inflammatory activities of extracts of the leaves of *Sphenocentrum jollyanum* Pierre. *J. Appl. Life Sci. Int.* **2017**, accepted.

29. Mbaka, G.O.; Adeyemi, O.O.; Adesina, S.A. Anti-diabetic activity of the seed extract of *Sphenocentrum jollyanum* and morphological changes on pancreatic beta cells in alloxan-induced diabetic rabbits. *J. Med. Med. Sci.* **2010**, *1*, 550–556.

30. Mbaka, G.; Adeyemi, O.; Osinubi, A.; Noronha, C.; Okanlawon, A. The effect of aqueous root extract of *Sphenocentrum jollyanum* on blood glucose level of rabbits. *J. Med. Plants Res.* **2009**, *3*, 870–874.

31. Mbaka, G.O.; Adeyemi, O.O.; Anunobi, C.C. Anti-hyperglycemic effects of ethanol leaf extract of *Sphenocentrum jollyanum* in normal and alloxan-induced diabetic rabbits. *Glob. J. Pharmacol.* **2008**, *2*, 46–51.

32. Alese, M.O.; Adewale, O.S.; Ijomone, O.M.; Ajayi, S.A.; Alese, O.O. Hypolipidemic and hypoglycemic activities of methanol extract of *Sphenocentrum jollyanum* on stretozocin induced diabetic Wistar rats. *Eur. J. Med. Plants* **2014**, *4*, 353–364. [CrossRef]

33. Mbaka, G.O.; Owolabi, M.A. Evaluation of Haematinic Activity and Sub chronic Toxicity of *Sphenocentrum jollyanum* (Menispermaceae) Seed Oil. *Eur. J. Med. Plants* **2011**, *1*, 140–152. [CrossRef]

34. Olorunnisola, O.S.; Afolayan, A.J. In Vivo antimalaria of methanol leaf and root extracts *Sphenocentrum jollyanum*. *Afr. J. Pharm. Pharmacol.* **2011**, *5*, 1669–1673. [CrossRef]

35. Mbaka, G.O.; Adeyemi, O.O.; Ogbonnia, S.O.; Noronha, C.C.; Okanlawon, O.A. The protective effect of ethanol root extract of *Sphenocentrum jollyanum* on the morphology of pancreatic beta cells of alloxan challenged rabbits. *J. Morphol.* **2011**, *28*, 37–45.

36. Olorunnisola, O.S.; Adetutu, A.; Fadahunsi, O.S. Anti-allergy potential and possible modes of action of *Sphenocentrum jollyanum* Pierre fruit extracts. *J. Phytopharm.* **2017**, *6*, 20–26.

37. Moody, J.O.; Robert, V.A.; Adeniji, J.A. Anti-viral effect of selected medicinal plants: *Diospyros bateri*, *D. monbutensis* and *Sphenocentrum jollyanum* on polio viruses. *Niger. J. Nat. Prod. Med.* **2002**, *6*, 4–6.

38. Moody, J.O.; Robert, V.A.; Hughes, J.A. Anti-viral activities of selected medicinal plantsand effect of extracts of Diospyrosmon butensis and *Sphenocentrum jollyanum* on cowpea mosaic viruses. *Pharm. Biol.* **2002**, *40*, 342–345. [CrossRef]

39. Woode, E.; Amidu, N.; Owiredu, K.; Boakye, G.; Ansah, C.; Duweijua, M. Antidepressant–Like effects of an ethanol extract of *Sphenocentrum jollyanum* Pierre Roots in Mice. *Int. J. Pharmacol.* **2009**, *5*, 22–29. [CrossRef]

40. Woode, E.; Duwiejua, M.; Ansah, C.; Kuffour, G.A.; Obiri, D.D.; Amidu, N. Effect of *Sphenocentrum jollyanum* in experimental mouse models of anxiety. In Proceedings of the 2nd Western Africa Network of Natural Products Research Scientists (WANNPRES), Elmina 32, Ghana, 1–4 August 2006; p. 32.

41. Woode, E.; Amidu, N.; Owiredu, K.; Boakye, G.; Laing, E.F.; Ansah, C.; Duweijua, M. Anxiogenic—Like effect of a root extract of *Sphenocentrum jollyanum* Pierre in Murine behaviour models. *J.Pharmacol. Toxicol.* **2009**, *4*, 91–108. [CrossRef]

42. Muko, K.N.; Ohiri, P.C.; Ezugwu, C.O. Antipyretic and analgesic activities of *Sphenocentrum jollyanum*. *Niger. J. Nat. Prod. Med.* **1998**, *2*, 52–53.

43. Owiredu, W.A.; Amidu, N.; Amissah, F.; Woode, E. The effects of ethanol extract of root of *Sphenocentrum jollyanum* Pierre on sexual behavior and hormonal levels in rodents. *J. Sci. Technol.* **2007**, *27*, 9–21.

44. Raji, Y.; Fadare, O.O.; Adisa, R.A.; Salami, S.A. Comprehensive assessment of the effect of *Sphenocentrum jollyanum* root extract on male albino rats. *Reprod. Med. Biol.* **2006**, *5*, 283–292. [CrossRef]

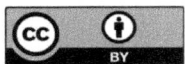

![medicines logo] *medicines*

MDPI

Article

Effects of Aqueous Extract of Three Cultivars of Banana (*Musa acuminata*) Fruit Peel on Kidney and Liver Function Indices in Wistar Rats

Chidi Edenta [1], Stanley I. R. Okoduwa [2,3,*] and Oche Okpe [4]

[1] Department of Biochemistry, Renaissance University, Ugbawka, Enugu State 402212, Nigeria; chidiedenta@gmail.com

[2] Directorate of Research and Development, Nigerian Institute of Leather and Science Technology, Zaria, Kaduna State 810221, Nigeria

[3] Infohealth Awareness Unit, SIRONigeria Global Limited, Abuja, Federal Capital Territory 900288, Nigeria

[4] Department of Biochemistry, Federal University of Agriculture, Makurdi, Benue State 970101, Nigeria; ocheking10@gmail.com

* Correspondence: siroplc@yahoo.com or stanley@sironigeria.com; Tel.: + 234-909-9640-143

Academic Editor: James D. Adams
Received: 25 September 2017; Accepted: 20 October 2017; Published: 23 October 2017

Abstract: Background: *Musa acuminata* fruit peels are used in the northern part of Nigeria for the treatment of hypertension and other cardiovascular related diseases. The effects of aqueous extracts of ripped fruit peel of three cultivars of *Musa acuminata* (*Saro, Ominni* and *Oranta*) on the hepatic and renal parameters of normal rats were examined. **Methods:** Fruit peel aqueous extracts (FPAE) of the 3 cultivars of Bananas (100 mg/kg b.w.) were administered by oral intubation (that is through esophageal cannula) to normal rats (140–180 g) for a period of 28 days. Blood samples were collected for determination of plasma aspartate amino transferase (AST), alanine amino transferase (ALT), alkaline phosphatase ALK-P), total protein, albumin, creatinine as well as urea. **Results:** From the results obtained, there were no significant ($p < 0.05$) changes in the ALK-P, AST, ALT, total protein and albumin among the experimental rats administered FPAE of the 3 cultivars of *Musa acuminata* when compared with the normal control group. There was a significant ($p < 0.05$) increase in the level of serum creatinine (in mg/dL) (1.53 ± 0.23) when compared to the normal control (0.72 ± 0.15), *Ominni* (0.92 ± 0.39) and *Oranta* (0.74 ± 0.22). Similarly, there was a significant ($p < 0.05$) increase in the level of serum urea (in mg/dL) of *Saro* (41.56 ± 4.68) when compared to the normal control (26.05 ± 0.73), *Ommini* (28.44 ± 2.43) and *Oranta* (26.10 ± 2.94). **Conclusion:** The findings reveal the *Saro* cultivar of *Musa acuminata* to be nephrotoxic and not a good potential drug candidate among the cultivars studied hence should be discouraged in the treatment of hypertension and other cardiovascular related diseases.

Keywords: banana; *Musa sapientum*; hepatotoxicity; nephrotoxicity; wistar rat; rats

1. Introduction

The liver plays a central role in the metabolism of drug, xenobiotics, protein synthesis and in maintaining biological equilibrium in organisms [1]. Although the liver is the target for most xenobiotics, the kidney usually shares in the burden of xenobiotic exposure, and the two organs carry out most of the biotransformation of xenobiotics [2]. Herbal drugs play a role in the management of various liver disorders, most of which speed up the natural healing processes of the liver [3]. Since ancient times, people have been exploring nature, particularly plants, in search of new drugs, and this has resulted in the use of a large number of medicinal plants with curative properties to treat various diseases [4]. The popularity and availability of the traditional remedies have generated concerns regarding the safety, efficacy and the responsibility of practitioners using traditional remedies [1]. Banana is one such plant that has gained popularity in treatment of various ailment.

Banana, generally known as *Musa sapientum*, is a familiar tropical fruit in the world. It originated mainly from intra- and inter-specific hybridizations between two wild diploid species, *M. acuminata* Colla ('A' genome) and *M. Balbisiana* Colla ('B' genome) [5]. Banana is a treelike perennial herb that grows 5–9 m in height, with a tuberous rhizome and a hard, long pseudo-stem. The inflorescence is big, with a reddish-brown bract, and is eaten as a vegetable. The ripe fruits are sweet, juicy and full of seeds, and the peel is thick [6,7]. Banana is the most popular fruit in industrialized countries. It is cultivated in over 130 countries as the second-most produced fruit after citrus [8,9]. It contributes approximately 17% of the world's total fruit production [8]. It is one of a good number of consumed fruits in tropical and subtropical regions of the world [10]. The scientific names of most cultivated bananas are *Musa acuminata*, *Musa balbisiana*, and *Musa × paradisiaca* for the hybrid *Musa acuminata × M. balbisiana*, depending on their genomic constitution. The old scientific name *Musa sapientum* is no longer used. The classification of cultivated bananas has long been a problematic issue for taxonomists. Bananas were originally placed into two species based only on their uses as food: *Musa sapientum* for dessert bananas and *Musa paradisiaca* for plantains. Series of papers published from 1947 onwards showed that *Musa sapientum* and *Musa paradisiaca* were actually cultivars, and were descendants of two wild seed-producing species, *Musa acuminata* and *Musa balbisiana*. In Nigeria, some of the most common edible banana cultivars include *Musa paradisiaca*, *Musa acuminata* (Cavendish banana) (MAC), and *Musa acuminata* (Red Dacca) (MAR) [11]. The cultivated varieties can present different genomic combinations: AA, AB, AAA, AAB, ABB, AAAA, AAAB, AABB and ABBB, diploids, triploids and tetraploids [5,12]. South-western Nigeria often blends the dried *Musa* spp. peels with the yam flour, as part of their stable foods [7].

The peels of bananas, constitute up to 35% of the ripe fruit, and are regarded as household and industrial food waste, being discarded in large quantities [13]. Taking a piece of banana peel and placing it on a wart, with the yellow side out, can be a natural alternative for killing off a wart; rubbing the affected area of a mosquito bite with the inside of a banana skin reduces swelling and irritation [14]. The peels of ripe bananas can be used to make a poultice for wounds, which is wrapped around an injury to reduce pain or swelling [15]. Banana tree has an important local and traditional value for treating anemic people. They are regarded as healthy food for children from around six months of age, because it does not produce cramps or diarrhea [16]. The ripe fruits/or pseudo-stems of bananas are used to treat diarrhea. The juice from *Musa* spp., is used to treat abdominal pain [16,17]. Unripe banana peels are used as a food source in scientific research, owing to their chemical composition, which was first described by [18]. Bioactive compounds such as alkaloids, anthocyanins, flavonoids, glycosides, phlobatannins, tannins, and terpenoids have been reported in banana peels, and these compounds have been shown to exert various biological and pharmacological effects (antibacterial, antihypertensive, antidiabetic, and anti-inflammatory activities) [16]. For the purpose of this research work, only three of the genomic combinations of *Musa acuminata* were used, which are the ones distributed within Nigeria. The cultivars are AA, AAB and ABB. Locally they are called *"Saro"*, *"Paranta/Oranta"* and *"Amina/Ominni"* respectively [12].

Musa acuminata fruit peels are used in the northern part of Nigeria for the treatment of hypertension and other cardiovascular related diseases [5]. Despite that several scientific studies that have validated the folkloric uses of different parts of the *banana*, there is no study in the open scientific literature that has provided scientific evidence for the claimed use of the peel of *Musa acuminata* in the management of cardiovascular related diseases. Additionally, no research has been done to determine the effects of its fruit peels on hepatic and renal parameters in rats. Therefore, this study was aimed at evaluating the effects of aqueous extract of three cultivars of *Musa acuminata* fruit peel on kidney and liver function indices in wistar rats.

2. Materials and Methods

2.1. Plant Sample Collection and Identification

The ripe banana fruit peels of the species (cultivars) *Saro, Oranta* and *Ominni* were collected from their natural habitat within Samaru (located on latitude: 11°9′55.3″ N and longitude: 7°39′5.84″ E), Zaria area of Kaduna State, Nigeria [19]. They were identified at the herbarium unit of the Biological Sciences Department, Ahmadu Bello University, Zaria Nigeria.

2.2. Experimental Protocols

Twenty wistar albino rats of both sexes weighing 140–180 g were purchased from the Faculty of Pharmaceutical Sciences, Ahmadu Bello University, Zaria-Nigeria. They were housed in polypropylene cages in a room where a congenital temperature was 27 °C ± 1 °C and 12 h light and dark cycles were maintained. The animals were allowed to acclimatize to the environment for fourteen days. During this period they were supplied with a commercial growers mash (Grand cereals limited, Jos, Nigeria) available in pellet form and water *ad libitum*.

2.3. Ethical Consideration

The study was approved on 18th September, 2014 by the Institutional animal care and use committee (Protocol number; AREC/EA14/273). All protocols were in accordance with the ethical committee guidelines that are in compliance with the National and International Laws and Guidelines for Care and Use of Laboratory Animals in Biomedical Research [20,21].

2.4. Period of Experimentation

The research was conducted between November 2014 and August 2015.

2.5. Preparation and Extractions of Plant Parts

The banana peels were air-dried in the laboratory for a period of two weeks and then made into powder by grinding and sieved with a mesh size of 0.05 mm. The banana peels aqueous extracts were prepared by soaking 300 g of the powder in 1500 mL (1:5) distilled water in a 2 L conical flask [22]. It was stirred and allowed to stand for 48 h. The extracts were thereafter filtered using filter paper. The filtrates were concentrated to dryness on a water bath set at 45 °C.

2.6. Acute Toxicity (LD_{50}) Test

The mean lethal dose of aqueous peel extracts of *Oranta, Ominni* and *Saro* of *M. acuminata* was determined in albino rats using the method described by Lorke [23]. The LD_{50} was conducted in a pilot study using 9 Wistar rats. The rats were randomly divided into 3 groups of 3 rats each and 10, 100, and 1000 mg/kg b.w., respectively, was administered orally. The animals were monitored for behavioral changes and mortality for 24 h. When no death was observed in any of the groups, 5 other groups were given 1250, 1500, 2000, 2500 and 5000 mg/kg b.w. of the extract and monitored for 24 h for changes in behavior and mortality. The LD_{50} is generally calculated as the geographical mean of the least lethal dose that killed a rat and the highest dose that did not kill a rat. Usually, the extract dose administered to the animal is either calculated as 1/10th of the observed acute toxicity test or extrapolated from the human dose. In this study, the reference body surface area of rat (0.02 m^2) [24] was multiplied by the maximum dose (5000 mg/kg b.w.) tested during the acute toxicity study [25]; that is, 0.02 × 5000 = 100.

2.7. Animal Grouping and Treatment

A total of 20 rats were used. The rats were divided into 4 groups of 5 rats each as follows:

Group I: Normal control received feed and distilled water only for 28 days.

Group II: Normal rats treated with *Saro* 100 mg/kg bw/day aqueous extract orally for 28 days.
Group III: Normal rats treated with *Ominni* 100 mg/kg bw/day aqueous extract orally for 28 days.
Group IV: Normal rats treated with *Oranta* 100 mg/kg bw/day aqueous extract orally for 28 days.

2.8. Blood Sample Collection

At the end of the experimental period, the rats were sacrificed by anesthesia using chloroform before sample collection through cardiac puncture. Blood was collected into EDTA bottles and centrifuged at 3500 rpm for 10 min and the clear sera aspirated off for biochemical evaluation.

2.9. Biochemical Analysis

Alanine aminotransferase (ALT) and aspartate aminotransferase (AST) were determined by monitoring the concentration of pyruvate hydrazone formed with 2,4, dinitrophenyl hydrazine and oxaloacetate hydrazone formed with 2,4-dinitrophenyl hydrazine respectively using Randox Diagnostic kits (Randox laboratories Ltd., Antrim, UK) [26]. Serum Creatinine and urea were assayed using standard procedures as described by Varley and Alan [27].

2.10. Statistical Analysis

Data obtained were expressed as mean ± SD. The data were analyzed using analysis of variance (ANOVA). The difference between the various extracts and animal groups were compared using the Duncan Multiple Range Test. The values of $p < 0.05$ were considered as statistically significant.

3. Results and Discussion

In the acute toxicity test study, no death was recorded even at a dose of 5000 mg/kg b.w. This signifies that the LD_{50} is greater than 5000 mg/kg b.w., hence there was nothing to present as results under this section. This observation was in agreement with the reports of Ezekwesili et al. [28]. According to the Hodge and Sterner [29] toxicity scale, *Musa acuminata* is said to be in the non-toxic herbal drug category [30]. The changes in serum liver marker enzymes and proteins of Wistar rats administered with extracts of *Musa acuminata* are shown in Tables 1 and 2, respectively. The results from this study show that there were no significant ($p > 0.05$) changes in the levels of aspartate amino transferase, alanine aminotransferase, alkaline phosphatase, total protein and albumin of all the extract-treated groups when compared to the normal control group. As shown in Table 3, there was a significant ($p < 0.05$) increase in the creatinine level of the group treated with the extract of *Saro* (1.53 ± 0.23) when compared with *Oranta* (0.74 ± 0.22), *Ominni* (0.92 ± 0.39) and normal control (0.72 ± 0.15) groups. Similarly, there was a significant ($p < 0.05$) increase in the level of serum urea of *Saro* (41.56 ± 4.68) when compared to the normal control (26.05 ± 0.73), *Ominni* (28.44 ± 2.43) and *Oranta* (26.10 ± 2.94) groups.

Table 1. Effect of *Musa acuminata* peels on some Serum Liver Marker Enzymes concentration in rats.

Groups ($n = 5$)	Serum ALK-P (U/L)	Serum ALT (U/L)	Serum AST (U/L)
NC	64.40 ± 15.93 [a]	43.53 ± 6.11 [a]	21.65 ± 5.77 [a]
N + OMN$_{100}$	36.80 ± 14.74 [a]	52.67 ± 8.32 [a]	25.01 ± 8.66 [a]
N + ORT$_{100}$	61.07 ± 10.16 [a]	41.33 ± 2.31 [a]	23.34 ± 7.64 [a]
N + SRO$_{100}$	46.03 ± 16.00 [a]	45.46 ± 9.24 [a]	26.67 ± 2.89 [a]

Values are means of five determination ± SD; [a] Values with different superscripts down the column are significantly different ($p < 0.05$); NC: Normal rats Control, N + SRO$_{100}$: Normal rats + Saro Extract (100 mg/kg), N + ORT$_{100}$: Normal rats + Oranta Extract (100 mg/kg), N + OMN$_{100}$: Normal rats + Ominni Extract (100 mg/kg), ALK-P: Alkaline Phosphatase, AST: Aspartate aminotransferase, ALT: Alanine aminotransferase.

Table 2. Effect of aqueous extracts of *Musa acuminata* peels on serum total protein and albumin concentration in rats.

Groups ($n = 5$)	Total Protein (g/L)	Albumin (g/L)
NC	56.95 ± 6.84 [a]	31.16 ± 6.31 [a]
N + OMN$_{100}$	64.46 ± 10.75 [a]	27.57 ± 2.07 [a]
N + ORT$_{100}$	65.23 ± 9.54 [a]	26.77 ± 3.30 [a]
N + SRO$_{100}$	60.25 ± 7.18 [a]	23.97 ± 3.74 [a]

Values are means of five determination ± SD. [a] Values with different superscripts down the column are significantly different ($p < 0.05$) NC: Normal rats Control, N + SRO$_{100}$: Normal rats + *Saro* Extract (100 mg/kg), N + ORT$_{100}$: Normal rats + *Oranta* Extract (100 mg/kg), N + OMN$_{100}$: Normal rats + *Ominni* Extract (100 mg/kg).

Table 3. Effect of aqueous extracts of *Musa acuminata* peels on serum creatinine and urea concentration in rats.

Groups ($n = 5$)	Creatinine (mg/dL)	Urea (mg/dL)
NC	0.72 ± 0.15 [a]	26.05 ± 0.73 [a]
N + OMN$_{100}$	0.92 ± 0.39 [a]	28.44 ± 2.43 [a]
N + ORT$_{100}$	0.74 ± 0.22 [a]	26.10 ± 2.94 [a]
N + SRO$_{100}$	1.53 ± 0.23 [b]	41.56 ± 4.68 [b]

Values are means ± SD of $n = 5$ determinations. [a] Values with different superscripts down the column are significantly different ($p < 0.05$), NC: Normal rats Control, N + SRO$_{100}$: Normal rats + *Saro* Extract (100 mg/kg), N + ORT$_{100}$: Normal rats + *Oranta* Extract (100 mg/kg), N + OMN$_{100}$: Normal rats + *Ominni* Extract (100 mg/kg).

The liver is the major organ of xenobiotic metabolism and detoxification, which makes it vulnerable to hepatotoxicity [31]. AST and ALT are key enzymes involved in the breakdown of amino acids into α-keto acid, which are routed for complete metabolism through the Krebs cycle and electron transport chain. They are regarded as precise biomarkers for liver damage. Also, changes in membrane-bound alkaline phosphatase (ALP) affects membrane permeability and produces derangement in the transport of metabolites [32]. Any damage on the liver results in the release of these marker enzymes into the system above a certain threshold [3]. From the results of our study as indicated in Table 1, it was observed that there were no significant changes ($p < 0.05$) in the levels of serum ALT, AST and ALP of all the extract treated groups when compared to normal control group. These observed insignificant ($p > 0.05$) changes are in accordance with good functioning of the liver. This implies that the peel extracts are not hepatotoxic. Concentrations of albumin and total protein in the serum can be used to assess the health status of the liver and can also be used to ascertain different type of liver damage [33–35]. The liver is the sole site for the synthesis of albumin, which makes up approximately 60% of serum protein concentration [36]. The present study revealed (Table 2) that there were no significant ($p > 0.05$) changes in total protein and albumin levels of the extract treated groups as compared to the normal control rats. The data obtained with respect to liver function indices indicate no cellular toxicity of the extracts on the liver of the experimental rats. However, as presented in Table 3, there was an increase in serum creatinine concentration (1.53 ± 0.23 mg/dL), reflecting a failed capacity of the kidney to effectively excrete creatinine. By inference, it implies that the ability of the two kidneys to effectively excrete creatinine, might have been exceeded. Serum creatinine and urea are common biomarkers for prediction of renal dysfunction, due to the fact that they are elevated considerably when there is a dysfunction of the kidney [33]. The level of serum creatinine usually doesn't rise until at least half of the nephrons of kidney are destroyed or damaged [37]. For differential diagnosis, simultaneous determination of serum creatinine along with urea is a standard practice; hence, serum urea was also estimated. Though urea is inferior to other markers, such as creatinine, blood urea is grossly influenced by other factors, such as diet and nutrition [38]. The marked significant increase in urea (41.56 ± 4.68) of *Saro* means that its intake may pose an undesirable effect on the kidney. Since the elevated levels of urea and creatinine are markers of kidney function [38,39], it then indicates that the extract of *Saro* peel cultivar may impair renal function at the comparative human dose levels.

4. Conclusions and Recommendation

The results from this study revealed that rats treated with the aqueous extracts of the three cultivars of *Musa acuminata* pose no threat to the liver. Conversely, aqueous extracts of *Saro* cultivars showed increase in the biomarkers of the kidney. Thus, intake of peel extracts of *M. acuminata*, particularly the *Saro* cultivar, as a drug might lead to potential kidney problems in the management and/or treatment of hypertension and other cardiovascular related diseases. At present, the exact mechanism of action of *M. acuminata* is not fully known. On this note, further investigations in this direction are needed for possible isolation and structural elucidation of the components of *M. acuminata*.

Acknowledgments: This research did not receive any specific grant from funding agencies in the public, commercial, or not-for-profit sectors. The authors express their warm appreciation to the management of SIRONigeria Global Limited, Abuja, for the English language proof editing and typesetting of the manuscript.

Author Contributions: S.I.R.O. and C.E. conceived and designed the experiments; C.E. performed the experiments; O.O. participated in the literature search. S.I.R.O. critically revised and review the manuscript for important intellectual content. All the enlisted authors contributed substantially to the success of the work reported and approve the final version for publication.

Conflicts of Interest: The authors declare no conflict of interest.

References

1. Sarkiyayi, S.; Aileru, A.E. Effect of methanol leaf extract of anogeissusleio carpus on gentamicin induced biochemical derangement in rats. *Direct Res. J. Health Pharmacol.* **2016**, *4*, 1–7.
2. Megaraj, V.; Ding, X.; Fang, C.; Kovalchuk, N.; Zhu, Y.; Zhang, Q.Y. Role of hepatic and intestinal p450 enzymes in the metabolic activation of the colon carcinogen azoxymethane in mice. *Chem. Res. Toxicol.* **2014**, *27*, 656–662. [CrossRef] [PubMed]
3. Rama, V.G.; Reddy, V.R.; Kumar, V.; Reddy, M.K. Hepatoprotectivity activity of medicinal plant extracts on Albino rats. *World J. Pharm. Sci.* **2016**, *5*, 1275–1284.
4. Ramesh, R.; Dhanaraj, T.S. Hepatoprotective effect of ethyl acetate extract of terminaliaarjuna root on hcb induced liver carcinogenes is in female albino wistar rats. *Int. J. Appl. Biol. Pharm. Technol.* **2016**, *7*, 190–199.
5. Edenta, C.; James, D.B.; Owolabi, O.A.; Okoduwa, S.I.R. Hypolipidemic effects of aqueous extract of three Cultivars of Musa sapientumfruit peel on poloxamer-407 induced hyperlipidemicwistar rats. *Int. J. Pharm. Sci. Res.* **2014**, *5*, 1046–1051.
6. Imam, M.Z.; Akter, S. *Musa paradisiaca* L. and *Musa sapientum* L. A Phytochemical and Pharmacological Review. *J. Appl. Pharm. Sci.* **2011**, *1*, 14–20.
7. Onasanwo, S.A.; Emikpe, B.O.; Ajah, A.A.; Elufioye, T.O. Anti-ulcer and ulcer healing potentials of Musa sapientum peel extract in the laboratory rodents. *Pharm. Res.* **2013**, *5*, 173–178. [CrossRef] [PubMed]
8. Food and Agriculture Organization (FAO). *FAOSTAT*; Food and Agriculture Organization: Geneva, Switzerland, 2013.
9. D'Hont, A.; Denoeud, F.; Aury, J.M. The banana (*Musa acuminata*) genome and the evolution of monocotyledonous plants. *Nature* **2012**, *488*, 213–217. [CrossRef] [PubMed]
10. Alkarkhi, A.F.M.; Ramli, S.; Yeoh, S.Y.; Easa, A.M. Physiochemical properties of banana peel flour as influenced by variety and stage of ripeness: Multivariate statistical analysis. *Asian J. Food Agro-Ind.* **2010**, *3*, 349–362.
11. Adedayo, B.C.; Oboh, G.; Oyeleye, S.I.; Olasehinde, T.A. Antioxidant and antihyperglycemic properties of three banana cultivars (*Musa* spp.). *Scientifica* **2016**. [CrossRef] [PubMed]
12. El-Khishin, D.A.; Belatus, E.L.; El-Hamid, A.A. Radwan, K.H. Molecular characterization of banana cultivars (*Musa* spp.) from Egypt using AFLP. *Res. J. Agric. Biol. Sci.* **2009**, *5*, 271–279.
13. Emaga, T.H.; Ronkart, S.N.; Robert, C.; Wathelet, B.; Paquot, M. Characterisation of pectins extracted from banana peels (Musa AAA) under different conditions using an experimental design. *Food Chem.* **2008**, *108*, 463–471. [CrossRef] [PubMed]
14. Kumar, K.P.S.; Bhowmik, D.; Duraivel, S.; Umadevi, M. Traditional and Medicinal Uses of Banana. *J. Pharm. Phytochem.* **2012**, *1*, 51–63.
15. Atzingen, D.A.; Gragnani, A.; Veiga, D.F.; Abla, L.E.; Mendonça, A.R.; Paula, C.A.; Juliano, Y.; Correa, J.C.; Faria, M.R.; Ferreira, L.M. Gel from unripe Musa sapientum peel to repair surgical wounds in rats. *Acta Cir. Bras.* **2011**, *26*, 379–382. [CrossRef] [PubMed]

16. Pereira, A.; Maraschin, M. Banana (*Musa* spp.) from peel to pulp: Ethnopharmacology, source of bioactive compounds and its relevance for human health. *J. Ethnopharmacol.* **2015**, *160*, 149–163. [CrossRef] [PubMed]
17. Abe, R.; Ohtani, K. An ethnobotanical study of medicinal plants and traditional therapies on Batan Island, the Philippines. *J. Ethnopharmacol.* **2013**, *145*, 554–565. [CrossRef] [PubMed]
18. Selema, M.D.; Farago, M.E. Trace element concentrations in the fruit peels and trunks of Musa paradisiaca. *Phytochemistry* **1996**, *42*, 1523–1525. [CrossRef]
19. Maduekwe, A.A.L.; Garba, B. Characteristics of the monthly averaged hourly diffuse irradiance at Lagos and Zaria, Nigeria. *Renew. Energy* **1999**, *17*, 213–225. [CrossRef]
20. National Research Council (NRC). *Guide for the Care and Use of Laboratory Animals*; National Academies Press: Washington, DC, USA, 2010.
21. Clark, J.D.; Gebhart, G.F.; Gonder, J.C.; Kneeling, M.E.; Kohn, D.F. The 1996 guide for care and use of laboratory animal animals. *ILAR J.* **1997**, *38*, 41–48. [CrossRef] [PubMed]
22. Okoduwa, S.I.R.; Umar, I.A.; James, D.B.; Habila, J.D. Evaluation of extraction protocols for anti-diabetic phytochemical substances from medicinal plants. *World J. Diabetes* **2016**, *7*, 605–614. [CrossRef] [PubMed]
23. Lorke, D. A new approach to practical acute toxicity testing. *Arch. Toxicol.* **1983**, *54*, 275–287. [CrossRef] [PubMed]
24. Nair, A.B.; Jacob, S. A simple practice guide for dose conversion between animals and human. *J. Basic Clin. Pharm.* **2016**, *7*, 27. [CrossRef] [PubMed]
25. Spielmann, H.; Genschow, E.; Liebsch, M.; Halle, W. Determination of the staring dose for acute oral toxicity (LD50) testing in the up and down procedure (UDP) from cytotoxicity data. *Altern. Lab. Anim.* **1999**, *27*, 957–966. [PubMed]
26. Reitman, S.; Frankel, S. A colorimetric method for the determination of serum glutamicoxaloacetic and glutamine pyruvic transaminases. *Am. J. Clin. Pathol.* **1957**, *28*, 56–63. [CrossRef] [PubMed]
27. Varley, H.; Alan, H.G. Tests in renal disease. In *Practical Clinical Biochemistry*; William Heinemann Medical Book Ltd.: London, UK, 1984; p. 1123.
28. Ezekwesili, C.N.; Ghasi, S.; Adindu, C.S.; Mefoh, N.C. Evaluation of the anti-ulcer property of aqueous extract of unripe Musa paradisiaca Linn peel in wistar rats. *Afr. J. Pharm. Pharmacol.* **2014**, *8*, 1006–1011.
29. Hodge, A.; Sterner, B. *Toxicity Classes*; Canadian Centre for Occupational Health Safety: Hamilton, ON, Canda, 2005. Available online: http://www.ccohs.ca/oshanswers/chemicals/id50.htm (accessed on 16 May 2016).
30. Ahmed, M. Acute Toxicity (Lethal Dose 50 Calculation) of Herbal Drug Somina in Rats and Mice. *Pharmacol. Pharm.* **2015**, *6*, 185–189. [CrossRef]
31. Ullah, I.; Khan, J.A.; Adhikari, A.; Shahid, M. Hepatoprotective effect of Monothecabuxifolia fruit against antitubercular drugs-induced hepatotoxicity in rats. *Bangladesh J. Pharmacol.* **2016**, *11*, 248–256. [CrossRef]
32. Okoduwa, S.I.R.; Umar, I.A.; James, D.B. Antidiabetic potential of occimum gratissimum leaf fraction in fortified diet fed streptozotocin-treated diabetic rats. *Medicines* **2017**, *4*, 73. [CrossRef] [PubMed]
33. Tierney, L.M.; Mcphee, S.J.; Papadakis, M.A. Current Medical Diagnosis and Treatment, International edition. In *New York: Lange Medical Books*; McGraw-Hill: New York, NY, USA, 2002; pp. 1203–1215.
34. Yakubu, M.T.; Bilbis, L.S.; Lawal, M.; Akanji, M.A. Evaluation of selected parameters of rat liver and kidney function following repeated administration of Yohimbine. *Biokemistri* **2003**, *15*, 50–56.
35. Nwaogu, L.A. Toxico-pathological evaluation of Citrulluscolocynthis seed and Pulp aqueous extracts on albino rats. *World J. Biol. Med. Sci.* **2016**, *3*, 76–85.
36. Khan, N.; Ahmed, M.; Khan, R.A.; Khan, S.; Gul, S. Evaluating the effect of Acacia modestaleaves extract on blood glucose, serum Lipids, liver and kidney functions in diabetic and non-diabetic rats. *Biomed. Nurs.* **2016**, *2*, 1.
37. Chukwuedozie, N.F. Evaluation of Time-Dependent Effects of a Leaf Extract of Spermacoceocymoideson Kidney Function. *J. Med. Biol. Sci. Res.* **2016**, *2*, 68–74.
38. Odoula, T.; Adeniyi, F.A.; Bello, I.S.; Subair, H.G. Toxicity studies on an unripe Caripa papaya aqueous extract; Biochemical and hematological effects in wistar albino rats. *J. Med. Plant Res.* **2007**, *1*, 1–4.
39. Grant, G.H. *Amino Acids and Proteins*; *Fundamentals of Clinical Chemistry*, 3rd ed.; Tietz, N.W., Ed.; WB Saunders Company: Philadelphia, PA, USA, 1987; pp. 328–329.

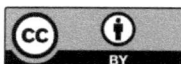

medicines

MDPI

Article

Medicinal Plants Used for Neuropsychiatric Disorders Treatment in the Hauts Bassins Region of Burkina Faso

Prosper T. Kinda [1], Patrice Zerbo [2], Samson Guenné [1], Moussa Compaoré [1], Alin Ciobica [3] and Martin Kiendrebeogo [1,*]

1   Laboratoire de Biochimie et Chimie Appliquées, Université Ouaga I-Pr Joseph KI-ZERBO,
    03 PB 7021 Ouagadougou 03, Burkina Faso; pros.kinda@hotmail.fr (P.T.K.); guesams@gmail.com (S.G.);
    mcompaore_3@yahoo.fr (M.C.)
2   Laboratoire de Biologie et écologie végétale, Université Ouaga I-Pr Joseph KI-ZERBO,
    03 BP 7021 Ouagadougou 03, Burkina Faso; patzerbo@yahoo.fr
3   "Alexandru Ioan Cuza" University of Iasi, Faculty of Biology, Department of Research, Carol I Avenue,
    No. 20A, Iasi 700505, Romania; alin.ciobica@uaic.ro
*   Correspondence: martinkiendrebeogo@yahoo.co.uk; Tel.: +226-7060-8590

Academic Editor: James D. Adams
Received: 16 December 2016; Accepted: 15 May 2017; Published: 19 May 2017

Abstract: Background: In Burkina Faso, phytotherapy is the main medical alternative used by populations to manage various diseases that affect the nervous system. The aim of the present study was to report medicinal plants with psychoactive properties used to treat neuropsychiatric disorders in the Hauts Bassins region, in the western zone of Burkina Faso. **Methods:** Through an ethnobotanical survey using structured questionnaire, 53 traditional healers (TH) were interviewed about neuropsychiatric disorders, medicinal plants and medical practices used to treat them. The survey was carried out over a period of three months. **Results:** The results report 66 plant species used to treat neuropsychiatric pathologies. Roots (36.2%) and leaves (29%) were the main plant parts used. Alone or associated, these parts were used to prepare drugs using mainly the decoction and the trituration methods. Remedies were administered via drink, fumigation and external applications. **Conclusions:** It appears from this study a real knowledge of neuropsychiatric disorders in the traditional medicine of Hauts Bassins area. The therapeutic remedies suggested in this work are a real interest in the fight against psychiatric and neurological diseases. In the future, identified plants could be used for searching antipsychotic or neuroprotective compounds.

Keywords: Neuropsychiatry; phytotherapy; traditional healers; Burkina Faso

1. Introduction

Nowadays, medicinal plant use in traditional therapy is increasing and diversifying. These plants were a precious patrimony for the humanity in general and particularly very important for developing countries people's healthcare and their subsistence [1]. They are invaluable resources for the great majority of rural populations in Africa, where more than 80% use them to ensure their primary healthcare [2]. According to the World Health Organization (WHO), neuropsychiatric disorders are a whole of "mental health problems", which are characterized by anomalies of the thought, emotions, behavior and relationship with others. These pathologies handicap the person concerned and assign people of its circle. Factors causing these disorders are essentially genetic, social, environmental and psychotropic drugs. Mental and neurological disorders represent 13% of the burden of total morbidity in the world [3]. Thirteen per cent to 49% of the world's populations develop neuropsychiatric disorders at some point in their life [4]. These pathologies affect all categories of person, race, sex and age [5]. Epilepsy is one of the most common neurological disorders. It affects more than 50 million persons in the world including 80% in developing countries [6]. High prevalence was observed in Africa where about 75% of patients do not receive adequate treatment [7]. The prejudices that surround neuropsychiatric diseases are causes of stigmatization of unwell persons who are often marginalized [3,8]. In Burkina Faso, 175‰ of the cases of disability are caused by neuropsychiatric disorders [6].

Many natural or synthetic psychoactive molecules such as neuroleptics, antidepressants, anxiolytics are used in modern medicine to treat these pathologies, particularly epilepsy, schizophrenia and the others psychotic disorders [8–10]. However, these modern treatments are expensive, complex and inaccessible for African populations in rural area [8,11]. Many of these psychoactive molecules have plant origins [12,13], which could justify plants use in the African traditional medicine to treat neuropsychiatric diseases [14,15]. In Burkina Faso, medicinal plants are widely used by peoples. Disapproved a long time after independences period for allopathic drugs [16], the government allowed in 1994 the traditional medicine practice. Since this time, it appeared a craze more and more growing for phytotherapy within the population, already predisposed to be directed there [17]. Moreover, many studies were undertaken to document plant species used in this therapy practice [18–22]. However, little research has approached the specific case of plants used to treat nervous system disorders in Burkina Faso. In the Hauts Bassins region, these pathologies were frequently denoted in psychiatric consultation [23,24]. Except Millogo's group works on "epilepsy and traditional medicine in Bobo-Dioulasso" [25], the traditional therapy of these pathologies is quoted only in other parallel studies. The present study aims to provide information about medicinal plants used to treat neuropsychiatric disorders in the Hauts Bassins region of Burkina Faso. It was necessary to report psychic and neurological disorders treated by traditional healers, medicinal plants and medical practices used for these treatments.

2. Materials and Methods

2.1. Study Area

The study was carried out in the Hauts Bassins region, located in western part of Burkina Faso (Figure 1). This area is known for its high phytogenetical and cultural diversity. Located at the West of Burkina Faso, between 9°21′N latitude and 2°27′W longitude, the Hauts Bassins region belongs to the phytogeographical sector of south-soudanien, characterized by average annual precipitations higher than 900 millimeters and average temperatures oscillating between 25 °C and 30 °C [26]. This sector is dominated by vegetable formations of savannas type timbered, arboreous or shrubby [27]. Several ethnics groups live in this area with a great diversity of cultural practices. The main spoken languages are Mooré (29.5%), Dioula (27.1%) and Bobo (18.8%) [28]. This region is characterized by a high number of traditional healers (TH) resulting from various ethnic groups. In addition to plant diversity and neuropsychiatric diseases frequency [24], the area was chosen because of the presence of various TH.

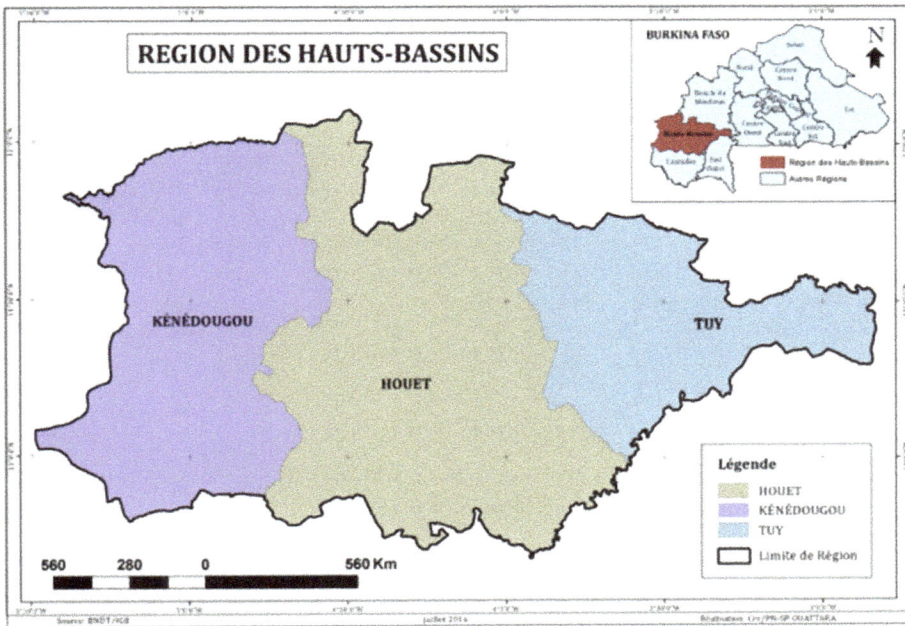

Figure 1. Study area localization (Hauts Bassins region of Burkina Faso).

2.2. Ethnobotanical Data Collection

The ethnobotanical survey was carried out during a three month period from October to December 2015. Data were collected using a structured interview with traditional healers (TH) who are organized in association. Through the association, a preliminary phone call was had with TH to inform them about objectives of the study. After that, an appointment were fixed with each one for individual interview. The approach was based on a dialogue using one of the three languages (Mooré, Dioula or French) to the TH choice. Pre-established questionnaires were used and a local person acting as a guide was necessary. Data were collected and transcribed on survey card-guides. It concerned medicinal plants used to treat the main psychiatric and neurological diseases such as epilepsy, mental disorders or madness, evils related to charm or witchcraft, hallucination or consciousness loss. These pathologies were reported to be more frequent in this area of Burkina Faso [24]. We gathered some of them because of their names in the local languages. Other collected information related to local names (in Mooré and/or Dioula) of plants, organs used of plants and medical practices such as drugs preparation and administration methods. Fifty-three TH including 35 men and 18 women, old from 31 to 82 years and having experience of plants use in traditional medicine were interviewed. Plants mentioned in the interview were collected in order to make the herbal constitution.

2.3. Data Analysis

Samples of plants collected were identified by botanists of the Ecology Department of University of Ouaga I-Pr Joseph Ki Zerbo (Burkina Faso). Then, voucher specimens were deposited in the herbarium of this University. The adopted nomenclature is that of "the tropical flora of Western Africa" [29], "medicinal plants and traditional medical practices in Burkina Faso" [30], "the catalogue of vascular plants of Burkina Faso" [31] and some enumerations of tropical Africa plants [32–34]. Plant parts used and medical practices were listed. Data were analyzed using SPSS software version 17.0 for window (SPSS Inc., Chicago, USA), and graphs were made on Excel of Office 2013.

3. Results

3.1. Plants Species Used

Sixty-six plant species including 51 woody and 15 herbaceous used to treat psychiatric and neurological diseases were identified. They belonged to 56 genera and 32 families (Table 1). Acacia and Ficus Genera were the most represented with 4 species each. The most represented families were Mimosaceae (8 species), Fabaceae (5 species) and Rubiaceae (5 species). Among these plants, the most used were showed on Table 2. A high use of Securidaca longepedunculata (45.3%), Calotropis procera (20.75%), Khaya senegalensis (20.75%), Allium sativum (20.75%), Daniellia oliveri (19%) and Annona senegalensis (17%) was observed by the majority of traditional healers (TH). Datura innoxia and Zanthoxlum zanthoxyloïdes were used by the oldest TH (more than 60 year old). Six species: S. longepedunculata, C. procera, K. senegalensis, A. senegalensis, Diospyros mespiliformis and Guiera Senegalensis were used to treat the main diseases targeted. Most of the plants were used alone and in association with other plants.

3.2. Plant Parts Used and Medical Practices

Various plant parts were used to prepare remedies (Figure 2a). Roots were mainly used (36.2%), followed by leaves (29%), mistletoes (9.3%) and stem barks (9%). Drugs preparation modes were the decoction (46.7%), the trituration (31%), the calcination (11.6%) and the aqueous maceration (10.7%) (Figure 2b). The drink (40.8%), the bath (33.8%), the fumigation (14.8%) and the massage (8.4%) are the main modes of administration (Figure 2c).

3.3. Neuropsychiatric Pathologies Treated

Diseases or regrouping diseases treated by traditional healers were registered in Table 3. From these results, hallucination or consciousness loss were most treated, followed by epilepsy, mental disorders and witchcraft or evils related to charm. In addition to these target pathologies, other cases such as insomnia and nerves diseases are also treated. Several plant species intervene in the treatment of each listed disorders. Thus, 37 plants were used to treat hallucination or consciousness loss, 32 to treat mental disorders, 31 to fight against epilepsy and 25 against diseases related to charm or witchcraft.

Table 1. Global information on plants used in various treatments.

Scientific Name (Genera and Specie)	Family	Local Name (Moore)	Local Name (Dioula)	Parts Used	Mode of Preparation	Mode of Administration	Pathologies Treated
Abrus precatorius L.	Fabaceae	Noraog-nini	Noronha	Fr	Cal	Mas	MA-MD
Acacia ataxacantha DC.	Mimosaceae	Kanguin péelga		Ro, Ba	Dec	Bat, Dri	EP
Acacia nilotica (L.) Willd. Ex Del.	Mimosaceae	Peg-nenga	Bangana	Ro	Dec	Bat, Dri	MA-MD
Acacia pennata (L.) Willd	Mimosaceae	Kanguinga		Ro	Dec	Bat, Dri	EP
Acacia sieberiana DC.	Mimosaceae	Gor-ponsego	Wenekassango	Le, Ro, Ba	Mac, Dec, Tri	Bat, Dri, Fum, Mas	MA-MD, HA-CL
Adansonia digitata L.	Bombacaceae	Tohèga	Sira-yiri	Le, Ro	Dec, Cal	Bat, Dri, Fum	MA-MD, HA-CL
Afzelia africana Smith ex Pers.	Caesalpiniaceae	Kankalga	Lingué, Lingué yiri	Le, Ro, Ba, Mi	Dec, Cal, Tri	Bat, Dri, Fum	MA-MD, HA-CL
Allium cepa L	Liliaceae	Zéyon	Djaba	Bu	Tri	Fum	EP
Allium sativum L.	Liliaceae	Layi	Bu	Bu	Dec, Cal, Tri	Bat, Dri, Fum, Pur, Mas	MA-MD, HA-CL
Annona senegalensis Pers.	Annonaceae	Barkudga	Mandé sunsun, Barkandé	Wp, Le, Ro, Ba	Dec, Cal, Tri	Bat, Dri, Fum, Mas	EP, MA-MD, CH-WI, HA-CL
Anogeissus leiocarpus (DC) Guill. & Perr.	Combretaceae	Siiga		Ba	Mac	Bat, Dri	HA-CL
Balanites aegyptiaca L.	Balanitaceae	Kyeguelga	Zéguenè	Le, Ro	Dec	Bat, Dri	MA-MD, CH-WI
Boscia senegalensis (Pers) Lam. ex Poir.	Capparidaceae	Lambwetga	Bere	Le, Ro	Dec	Bat, Dri	EP
Boswellia dalzielii Hutch	Burseraceae	Gondregneogo, Kondregneogo		Ro, Ba	Mac, Dec, Tri	Bat, Dri, Fum	HA-CL
Calotropis procera (Ait) Ait. F.	Asclepiadaceae	Putrepuuga	Fogofogo	Wp, Le, Ro, Mi, La	Mac, Dec, Tri	Bat, Dri, Fum, Ing	EP, MA-MD, CH-WI, HA-CL
Ceiba pentandra (L.) Gaertn	Bombacaceae	Gounga	Bana-yiri	Ro	Cal	Dri	EP
Cissus quadrangularis L.	Vitaceae	Wob-Zanré	Oulouyoroko	St	Cal	Dri	EP
Citrus aurantifolia (Christm.) Swingle	Rutaceae	Lembur-tiiga	Laimbourou	Fr, Mi	Mac, Dec, Cal	Bat, Dri, Mas	MA-MD, CH-WI, HA-CL
Crateva adansonii DC.	Capparidaceae	Kalguem-tohèga		Le	Dec	Dri	CH-WI
Cymbopogon giganteus Chiov.	Poaceae	Kuwaré	Tiékala	Le, Ro	Dec	Dri	MA-MD, HA-CL
Cymbopogon proximus (Hochst ex A. Rich) Stapf	Poaceae	Soompiiga		Wp, Ro	Cal	Dri	CH-WI
Dalbergia melanoxylon Guill. & Perr.	Fabaceae	Guirdiandèga		Ro	Mac	Fum	MA-MD, HA-CL
Daniellia oliveri (Rolfe) Hutch et Dalz	Caesalpiniaceae	Aoga, Anwga	sana, sana yiri	Le, Ro, Ba, Mi	Mac, Dec, Cal, Tri	Bat, Dri, Fum	MA-MD, CH-WI, HA-CL
Datura innoxia Mill.	Solanaceae	Barassé, Zèebla	Alomoukaïkaï	Le, Fr	Cal	Dri, Mas	MA-MD,CH-WI, HA-CL,IN,ND
Detarium microcarpum Guill. & Perr.	Caesalpiniaceae	kagadèga	Tamakouma	Le, Ro	Dec	Bat, Dri	EP; CH-WI, HA-CL
Diospyros mespiliformis Hochst ex A. DC	Ebenaceae	Gaaka, Gaanka	Sounsoun, Sounsounfi	Le, Ro	Mac, Dec	Bat, Dri	EP; MA-MD, CH-WI, HA-CL
Entada africana Guill. & Perr.	Mimosaceae	Séonego	Ro	Ro	Dec	Bat, Dri	EP
Faidherbia albida (Del.) A. Chev.	Mimosaceae	Zaanga	Balanzan, Balàzä	Le, Ro	Dec	Bat, Dri	CH-WI

Table 1. *Cont.*

Scientific Name (Genera and Specie)	Family	Local Name (Mooré)	Local Name (Dioula)	Parts Used	Mode of Preparation	Mode of Administration	Pathologies Treated
Ficus ingens (Miq.) Miq.	Moraceae	Kunkwiga		Ro	Dec	Dri	EP
Ficus iteophylla Miq.	Moraceae	Kunkwi-péelga	Djetigui faaga, Diatiguifaga	Le, Ro, Ba	Mac, Dec	Bat, Dri	EP, MA-MD, HA-CL
Ficus sycomorus L.	Moraceae	Kankanga	Toro, toro yiri	Le, Ro, Mi	Dec, Tri	Bat, Dri	EP, HA-CL
Ficus vallis-choudae Delile	Moraceae		Torossaba, Toroba	Le, Ro	Dec	Bat, Dri	EP
Flueggea virosa (Roxb ex. Willd) Voigt.	Euphorbiaceae	Sugdin-daaga	Balabala, Bala-bala	Le, Ro	Dec	Bat, Dri	CH-WI
Gardenia sp.	Rubiaceae	Subudga, Lambrezunga	Bure, Buré yiri	Wp, Le, St, Ro	Dec, Cal	Bat, Dri	EP, CH-WI, HA-CL
Guiera senegalensis J.F. Gmel	Combretaceae	Wilin-wiiga	Koungoué, Kungoué	Wp, Le, Ro, Mi	Dec, Cal, Tri	Bat, Dri	EP, MA-MD, CH-WI, HA-CL
Hygrophila senegalensis (Nees) T. Anderson	Acanthaceae		Kelebetokalla, Klebato-yiri	Le	Mac, Dec	Bat, Dri	EP
Hyptis spicigera Lam.	Lamiaceae	Rung-rungui	Timitimini.	Wp	Dec	Bat, Dri	EP
Indigofera tinctoria L.	Fabaceae	Garga		Le	Tri	Pur	HA-CL
Khaya senegalensis (Desr) A. Juss	Meliaceae	Kuka	Diala, Djala	Le, Ba, Mi	Mac, Dec, Cal, Tri	Bat, Dri, Fum	EP, MA-MD, CH-WI, HA-CL
Lannea acida A. Rich	Anacardiaceae	Labtulga		Le, Ro, Ba	Dec, Tri	Bat, Dri	EP, HA-CL
Leptadenia hastata (Pers.) Decne	Asclepiadaceae	Lelongo	Kosafla	Wp, Le, St, Ro	Dec	Bat, Dri	MA-MD, HA-CL
Mitracarpus villosus (SW.) DC.	Rubiaceae	Yod-péelga		Wp	Tri	Fum	MA-MD
Mitragyna inermis (Willd) O. Ktze	Rubiaceae	Yiilga	Djou, Diou, Jun, dioum	Wp, Le, Ro	Dec, Tri	Bat, Dri, Fum	EP, MA-MD, HA-CL
Moringa oleifera Lam.	Moringaceae	Arzan-tiiga	Masa yiri	Ro	Dec	Bat, Dri, Fum	MA-MD
Nicotiana rustica L.	Solanaceae	Kinkirs taba, Waamb-tabré	Flavourou	Le	Tri	Fum	HA-CL
Nicotina tabacum L.	Solanaceae	Taba	Kotaba	Le	Cal	Dri, Mas	CH-WI
Ocimum americanum L.	Lamiaceae	Yulin-gnu-raaga	Sukuola	Wp, Le	Dec, Tri	Bat, Fum	EP, HA-CL
Ocimum basilicum L.	Lamiaceae	Yulin-gnuuga	Sukuola-sina	Le	Tri	Fum	HA-CL
Parkia biglobosa (Jacq.) R. BR. ex G. Don. F	Mimosaceae	Roaaga	Néré	Le, Ro, Mi	Mac, Dec	Bat, Dri	EP, MA-MD, CH-WI
Pennisetum americanum Stapf	Poaceae	Kazui	Sagnon	Fr	Tri	Pur	EP, CH-WI
Pericopsis laxiflora (BentH ex Bak.) V. Meeawen	Fabaceae	Taankomiiga	Kolo-kolo, Kolokolo yiri	Le, St	Dec, Tri	Bat, Dri, Fum	MA-MD, HA-CL
Prosopis africana (Guill. Perr. & Rich) Taub.	Mimosaceae	Duanduanga, yamagui	Goulé, Gouélé	Ro, Fr	Dec, Cal	Bat, Dri	CH-WI
Pseudocedrela kotschyi (Schweinf.) Harms	Meliaceae	Siguedré		Le	Dec	Bat, Dri	MA-MD, HA-CL
Saba senegalensis (A. DC) Pichon	Apocynaceae	wédga	Zaban yiri	Ro	Dec	Bat	HA-CL
Sclerocarya birrea (A. Rich) Hochst	Anacardiaceae	noabga		Le, Ba	Dec	Dri	EP
Scoparia dulcis L.	Scrophulariaceae	Kafremaandé		Wp	Tri	Fum	MA-MD, HA-CL

Table 1. *Cont.*

Scientific Name (Genera and Specie)	Family	Local Name (Mooré)	Local Name (Dioula)	Parts Used	Mode of Preparation	Mode of Administration	Pathologies Treated
Securidaca longepedunculata Fresen	Polygalaceae	Pelga	Djoro, Diouro	Le, Ro, Ba	Mac, Dec, Cal, Tri	Bat, Dri, Fum, Pur, Mas	EP, MA-MD, CH-WI, HA-CL
Sterculia setigera Del.	Sterculiaceae	Ponsemporgo, Putermuka	Congo-sera, Kongossira	Ro, Mi	Dec	Bat, Dri	EP
Strychnos spinosa Lam.	Loganiaceae	Katrepoaga, Katerpoagha	Kogobaranie, Fouflé barani	Fr	Tri	Ing	CH-WI
Stylosanthes erecta P. Beauv.	Fabaceae	Sakwisabelga		Wp	Cal	Mas	CH-WI
Tamarindus indica L.	Caesalpiniaceae	Pusga	Ntomi, Toni	Le, Ro, Fr, Mi	Mac, Dec, Tri	Bat, Dri, Fum	EP, MA-MD, HA-CL
Vitellaria paradoxa C.F. Gaertn	Sapotaceae	Taanga	Schi yiri, Si yiri	Le, Ro, Mi	Dec, Tri	Bat, Dri, Fum	MA-MD, CH-WI, HA-CL
Vitex doniana Sweet	Verbenaceae	Aadga	Koto	Le, Ro	Dec	Bat, Dri	MA-MD
Ximenia americana L.	Olacaceae	Leenga		Le, Ro	Dec, Cal	Bat, Dri	MA-MD, CH-WI, HA-CL
Zanthoxylum zanthoxyloïdes Lam. Zep et Timl	Rubiaceae	Rapeoka	Wo	Ro, Ba	Tri	Dri, Fum, Mas	EP, MA-MD, HA-CL, IN
Zizyphus mauritiana Lam.	Rhamnaceae	Mugunuga	Tomonon	Le, Ro, Mi	Dec, Tri	Bat, Dri	EP, HA-CL

Part used: Whole plants (Wp); Leaves (Le); Stems (St); Roots (Ro); Barks (Ba); Flowers (Fl); Fruits (Fr); Mistletoes (Mi); Bulbs (Bu); Latex (La). **Mode of preparation:** Maceration (Mac); Decoction (Dec); Calcination (Cal); Trituration (Tri). **Mode of administration:** Bath (Bat); Drink (Dri); Fumigation (Fum); Purging (Pur); Massage (Mas); Ingestion (Ing). **Pathologies:** Epilepsy (EP); Madness or Mental Disorders (MA-MD); Charm or Witchcraft (CH-WI); Hallucination or Consciousness Loss (HA-CL); Insomnia (IN); Nerves diseases (ND).

Table 2. Main plants used, rate and age of TH user, rate of treated diseases and type of use.

Plants	User TH Rate (%)	Average Age of TH	Treated Diseases Rate (%)	Use Alone or Associated
Acacia sieberiana DC.	7.5	45	75	alone
Afzelia africana Smith ex Pers.	11.3	42	75	alone, associated
Allium sativum L.	20.75	57.5	50	associated
Annona senegalensis Pers.	17	55.5	100	alone, associated
Calotropis procera (Ait) Ait. F.	20.75	57	100	alone, associated
Citrus aurantifolia (Christm.) Swingle	7.5	51	75	associated
Daniellia oliveri (Rolfe) Hutch. et Dalz.	19	45.5	75	alone, associated
Datura innoxia Mill.	13.2	60.5	75	alone, associated
Detarium microcarpum Guill. et Perr.	5.7	39	75	associated
Diospyros mespiliformis Hochst ex A. DC.	13.2	39	100	alone, associated
Ficus iteophylla Miq.	7.5	39	75	alone, associated
Guiera senegalensis J.F. Gmel.	13.2	50	100	alone, associated
Khaya senegalensis (Desr) A. Juss	20.75	47	100	alone, associated
Mitragyna inermis (Willd) O. Ktze	7.5	35.5	75	alone, associated
Parkia biglobosa (Jacq.) R. BR. ex G. Don.F	7.5	48	75	alone
Securidaca longepedunculata Fresen	45.3	48	100	alone, associated
Tamarindus indica L.	11.3	46	75	associated
Ximenia americana L.	5.7	46	75	alone, associated
Zanthoxylum zanthoxyloïdes Lam. Zep &Timl	7.5	60	75	alone, associated
Ziziphus mauritiana Lam.	5.7	47	75	alone, associated

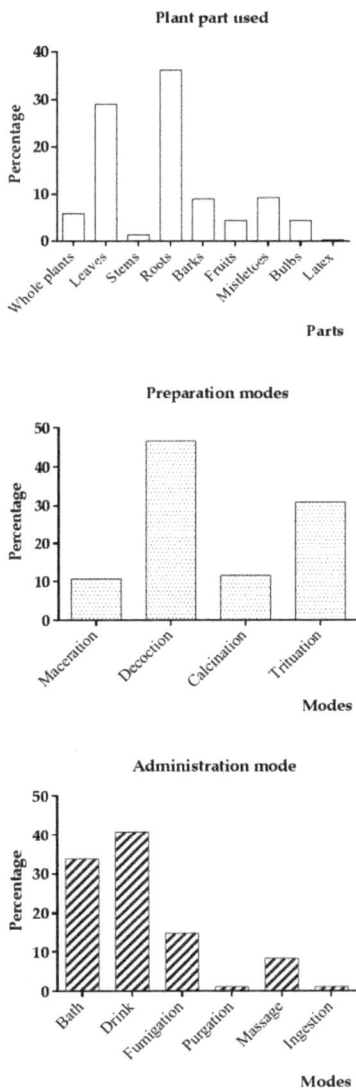

Figure 2. Plant parts used, modes of preparation and administration of remedies.

Table 3. Pathologies treated, traditional healers (TH) rate and medicinal plants used.

Pathologies			Treating TH Rate (%)	Number of Plants Used
English Name	**Local Name (*Mooré*)**	**Local Name (*Dioula*)**		
Epilepsy	*Kisinkindou*	*Cricromansian*	49	31
Hallucination or Consciousness loss	*Ningyilinga, sobgré*	*Djina bana*	79.2	37
Insomnia	*Gueim Baansé*	*Sinōgōtan ya*	3.8	2
Mental disorders or Madness	*Guimdo, Jougkolgo*	*Faatō ya*	47.2	32
Nerves diseases	*Guiin Baansé*	*Fassadjourou bana*	3.8	1
Witchcraft or Charm diseases	*Rabsgo, Soondo*	*Soubaga ya*	35.8	25

4. Discussion

Traditional medicine practice in Hauts Bassins area is rich and diversified. The most often treated neuropsychiatric disorders are hallucination, epilepsy and mental disorders, respectively treated by 79.2%, 49% and 47.2% of traditional healers (TH). These data correspond to those of other works [7,25,35], which revealed that these pathologies are well-known and treated in the traditional medicine of many African countries.

Sixty-six (66) plant species belonging to various families used in the treatment of neuropsychiatric disorders were listed. This result testifies TH knowledge about plants diversity of this area and their therapeutic virtues. Similar results were observed by previous studies [19,21] which showed that local populations of Burkina Faso were known to profit from the best part of biodiversity in traditional medicine. More than 77% of plants identified are ligneous. This rate could be justified by the relative abundance of these species in the phytogeographical sector of this area, and their availability during all the year. These results were in the same order with those of Traoré's group in the province of Comoé [36], Olivier's group on "Dozo" traditional healers [21] and Zerbo's group in western area [22], which indicates a prevalence of ligneous use in the pharmacopeia of this zone of Burkina Faso. *S. longepedunculata, C. procera, K. senegalensis, A. sativum, D. oliveri, A. senegalensis* were identified as the main species used and *D. innoxia, Z. zanthoxyloïdes* were only used by older TH. They were cited like plant species intervening in the treatment of neuropsychiatric disorders in others African countries [8,35,37]. According to many authors, all these plants have phytochemical components with effects on the nervous system [38,39]. They contain alkaloids, terpenoids, steroids, flavonoids, tannins, saponins and cardiac glycosides (Table 4). These chemical constituents were considered as the main bioactive compounds of medicinal plants [30,40,41]. *C. procera* root bark used in the treatment of anxiety, epilepsy, and madness contain alkaloids such as α-amyrin, β-amyrin, while its leaf and its latex possess cardenolides such as calactin, calotoxin, calotropin and uscharin [42,43].

These chemical contents could be responsible of the traditional use of this plant. Besides, *C. procera* extracts were reported to possess significant anticonvulsant and analgesic properties [42,44]. Tropanic alkaloids as scopolamin, atropin, hyoscinian isolated in *D. innoxia* are known for their anticholinergic effects. They act as acetylcholin antagonists [15]. Scopolamine is an antimuscarinic agent used as analgesic and relaxant [45]. Anticholinergic and antimuscarinic effect of these compounds could explain in part Datura use in mental diseases treatement. Securidine, an alkaloid isolated from *S. longepedunculata* root, has a stimulating effect on the spinal cord. Used in a non-toxic dose, it influenced the function of the autonomic nervous system [46]. Some flavonoids were reported to possess anxiolytic effects and neuroprotective activities; they are capable of binding to GABAA receptors with significant affinity [47]. As examples, 6-methylapigenin is a benzodiazepine binding site ligand and 2S(-)-hesperidin has sedative and sleep-enhancing properties [48]. Quercetin significantly decreased the brain ischemic lesion [49]. Hesperidin was identified in *C. aurantifolia* and *Z. zanthoxyloïdes*, while apigenin was isolated from *S. longepedunculata* and Quercetin in most of plants listed in this study (Table 4).

These bioactive compounds could explain plants efficacy in the treatment of neuropsychiatric diseases [50,51]. Mechanisms through which these compounds act on the central nervous system are various including regulation of neurotransmitters activity [52–54]. However, benefical activities of these plants do not occult their toxic effects. Indeed, they have also cytotoxic and cardiotoxic effects [42]. Securinine in the range 5–30 g/kg act like strychnine, causing spasms and death by respiratory arrest [46]. Tropanic alkaloids are potential neurotoxic agents [15]. Therefore, a controlled use of these plants should be promoted.

Table 4. Phytochemical constituents and pharmacological properties of main plants used.

Plants	Pharmacological Properties	Phytochemical Constituents	Chemical Compounds Identified
Acacia sieberiana DC.	Inhibition of acetylcholinesterase, anti-inflammatory [55].	Alkaloids, cyanogenic glucoside, tannins, terpenoids, Saponins, Flavonoids, essential oils, Cardiac glycosides, steroid, resins [56–58].	Dihydroacacipetalin; acacipetalin [56]. Manganese; calcium; magnesium; cupper, iron, zinc, nickel [57].
Afzelia africana Smith ex Pers.		Alkaloids, tannins, saponins, fiber, flavonoids, cyanides, beta-carotenes, cyanogenic glycosides, terpenoids, steroids, anthocyanins [59–61].	Sodium; potassium; calcium; magnesium; phosphorus; iron; zinc; vitamins A, C, E, B1, B2, B6, B12 [59,62].
Allium sativum L.	Stimulant, antioxydant, anti-inflammatory, antimicrobial, fungicidal, antibacterial, anticancerous, chemopreventive, anti-tumoral, antidiabetic [63–65].	Alkaloids, phenolics, flavonoids, essential oils [64,66,67]	Trisulphide-di-2-propenyl; artumerone; tetrazolo [1,5-b] pyridazine; 2-hydroxyethyl ethyl disulfide; cyclic octa-atomic sulphur [66]. Allin; allicin [63]. Diallyl trisulfide; diallyl disulfide; methyl allyl trisulfide [65]. Diallyl monosulfide; trisulfide méthyl-2-propenyl; diméthyl tétrasulfide [68].
Annona senegalensis Pers.	Anticonvulsant, anxiolytic, sedative, antibacterial, anti-inflammatory, cytotoxic, antioxydant, anti-nociceptive, antivenenous [15,69].	Alkaloids, flavonoids, saponins, sterols, flavonols, triterpenes, diterpenoids phenols, antraquinones, anthocyanes, coumarines [15,70]	1,2-benzenediol; butylate hydroxytoluene; methylcarbamate; n-hexadecanoique acid; hexadecane; acide oleique; etracosane; 9-octylheptadecane; heneicosane; 13-octadecadien-1-ol; octadecanoique acid; 9,17-octadecandienal; pentadecane; tetratriacontaue; squalene [71]. Kaurenoic acid [69]
Calotropis procera (Ait) Ait. F.	Anticonvulsant, analgesic, anti-inflammatory,antitumoral, hepatoprotective, antioxidant, spasmolytic, cytotoxic, cardio-stimulantg, lipase inhibitory, anti-apoptotic [42,72–74].	Alkaloids, cardenolides, triterpenes, flavonoids, sterols, saponins, diterpenes, resines, tannins, steroides [43,75].	Calactin; calotropagenin; calotropin; calotoxin; uscharin; syriogenin, afrogenin [42,43]. Flavonoid 5-hydroxy-3,7-dimethoxyflavone-4′-O-β-glucopyranoside; 3-O-rutinosides of quercetin; kaempferol; isorhamnetin [75]. Cholin; uscharin; uscharidin; voruscharidin; α-amyrine; β-amyrine [30,76].
Citrus aurantifolia (Christm.) Swingle	Antioxidant, anti-inflammatory, fungicidal, antibacterial [77–79].	Essential oils, glucosides, carotenoids, flavonoïds [67,77].	α-pinene; camphene; sabinene; β-pinene; myrcene; Δ3-carene; limonene; (Z)-β-ocimene; α-terpinene; γ-terpinene ; terpinolene; linalool; citronnelal; isocamphene; borneol; terpinen-4-ol; myrtenal; δ-cadinene; caryophyllen oxide; α-eudesmol; myrcene; p-cymene; benzoic acid; α-cedrene; α-bergamotene; α-bisabolene [77–79]. Hespéridine, vitamine C [67].
Daniellia oliveri (Rolfe) Hutch. et Dalz.	Analgesic, antihistaminic, relaxant, anti-inflammatory, antimicrobial, antidiabetic, antispasmodic, antipyretic, antidiarrhoeal [80–82]	Alkaloids, saponosides, flavonoids, glycosides, diterpenoids, sitosterol, coumarines, antracenosides, tanins, hétérosides cardiotoniques, trierpènes, Sterols [8,81,82].	Rutin; quercitin-3/-O-methyl-3-O-a-rhamnopyranosyl-(→)-β-D-glucopyranoside (Narcissin); quercitrin; quercimeritrin [80,81].

Table 4. *Cont.*

Plants	Pharmacological Properties	Phytochemical Constituents	Chemical Compounds Identified
Datura innoxia Mill.	Hallucinogen, analgesic, hypnotic, narcotic, anti-cholinergic, antiparkinsonien, sedative, cytotoxic, aphrodisiac, antispasmodic, antiemetic, anti-aflatoxine, anti-bradycardic, anti-inflammatory, anti-dizziness, antitumor [83–85]	Alkaloids tropanics [83,86].	Hyoscyamine; scopolamine; tropinone; tropine; pseudotropine; scopoline; scopine; 3-acetoxytropane; 3-acetoxy-6-hydroxytropane; cuscohygrine; aposcopolamine; 3(α′),6-ditigloyloxytropane; 3(β′),6-ditigloyloxytropane; 3-(′-acetoxytropoyloxy)-tropane; 3,6-Ditigloyloxy-7-hydroxytropane; 7-hydroxyhyoscyamine; 6-hydroxyhyoscyamine; 3-tropoyloxy-6-isovaleroyloxytropane; 6-tigloylhyoscyamine; luteoline [83,85,86].
Detarium microcarpum Guill. et Perr.		Alkaloid, fibers, tannins, saponins, flavonoids, cyanides, beta carotenes, cyanogenic glycosides, terpenoids, sterols, anthocyanines [59,61].	Calcium; phosphorus; iron; zinc; vitamins A, E [59].
Diospyros mespiliformis Hochst ex A. DC.	Antioxydant, astringent, spasmolytic, antibacterial, homeostatic [87].	Alkaloids, polyphenols, flavonoids, anthraquinones, tannins, triterpenes, saponins, saponosides, anthocyanes, anthracenosides, steroids [87,88].	
Ficus iteophylla Miq.	Analgesic, anti-inflammatory, antibacterial [89]	Steroids, furanocoumarines, flavonoids glycosides [80,89]	3β-cholest-5-ene-3, 23diol; 24 ethyl cholest-5-ene- 3β-ol [89].
Guiera senegalensis J.F. Gmel.	Psychoactive, detoxicant, anti-plasmodial, antimicrobial, antifungal, antioxydant, anticancerous, antiviral, [90,91].	Alkaloids, flavonoids, triterpenes, tannins, cardenolides, anthracene, coumarines, sterols, saponosides [91,92].	
Khaya senegalensis (Desr) A. Juss	Anticonvulsant, Anxiolytic, sedative, antioxydant, anti-tumoral, chemopreventive, anti-inflammatory [15,93–95].	Alkaloids, saponins, tannins, triterpenes, flavonoids, glucosides, carbohydrate, phylates, oxalates, triterpenoids [15,94,95].	Gedunin; methyl-angolensate; methyl-6-hydroxyangolensate [96]. Catechin; rutin; quercetin rhamnoside; procyanidins [97]. Fissinolide; 2,6-dihydroxyfissinolide; methyl 3b-acetoxy-6-hydroxy-1-oxomeliac-14-enoate [98]. Magnesium, calcium, potassium, sodium, zinc, iron, manganese, lead, chromium [94].
Mitragyna inermis (Willd) O. Ktze	Anticonvulsant, cardiovascular affects, antibacterial, antiplasmodial, anti-diabetic [99–101].	Alkaloids, polyphenols, sterols, polyterpenes, quinones, tannins, saponins, flavonoids, saponosides [99,100,102].	Rhynchophylline; isorhynchophylline; corynoxeine; isocorynoxeine; ciliaphylline; rhyncociline; isospcionoxeine; 9-methoxy-3-epi-α-yohimbine [103]. 27-nor-terpenoid glucoside [104,105].
Parkia biglobosa (Jacq.) R. BR. ex G. Don. F	Antibacterial, antifungal, antioxidant, antihyperlipidemic, cardioprotective [106–108].	Alkaloids, cardiac glycosides, tannins, steroids, tannins, alkaloids, flavonoids, saponins, terpenes, glycosides [106,109].	

Table 4. *Cont.*

Plants	Pharmacological Properties	Phytochemical Constituents	Chemical Compounds Identified
Securidaca longepedunculata Fresen	Anticonvulsant; antidepressant, anxiolytic, antioxydant, anti-nociceptive, cytotoxic, antivenomous, antibactérial, aphrodisiac, sedative, [110–112].	Alkaloids, saponosides, flavonoids, phenols, xanthones, anthraquinones, essential oils [113–115].	Gallic acide; quercetin; cafeic acid; chlorogenic acid; epicatechin; p-coumaric acid; cinnamic acid; rutin; apigenin [82] Phelandrene; pinene; z-sabinol; limonene; p-cymene [110] Securinin [116,117]. Muchimangine E, muchimangine F [118].
Tamarindus indica L.	Analgesic, antinociceptive, antivenin, hepatoprotective, anti-inflamatory, anti-helminthic, antioxydant, antibacterial [119–121].	Alkaloids, saponins, glycosides, tannins, terpenoids, flavonoids, coumarins, naphthoquinones, anthraquinones, xanthonones [121–124].	C-glycosidesorientin; vitexin; isoorientin; isovitexin; tartaric acid; malic acid [120]. Limonene; methyl salicylate; pyrazine; alkylthiazole; calcium; iron; zinc; vitamins B and C [125].
Ximenia americana L.	Anti-plasmodiale, antioxidant, anticancer, antineoplastic, antitrypanosomal, antirheumatic, antioxidant, analgesic antipyretic [90,126,127].	Alkaloids, anthraquinones, cardiac glycosides, flavonoids, pylobatannins, sapponins, tannins, terpenoids, isoprenoids, triterpenes, sesquiterpenes, quinones [126–128].	Norisoprenoid isophorane; ximenynic acid; methyl-14,14-dimethyl-18-hydroxyheptatracont-27,35-dienoate; dimethyl-5-Methyl-28,29-dihydroxydotriacont-3,14,26-triendioate; 10Z,14E,16E-octadeca-10,14,16-triene-12-ynoic acid, tariric acid; β-sitosterol; oleanene palmitates [127,129,130] .
Zanthoxylum zanthoxyloides Lam. Zep &Timl	Antiplasmodial, vasorelaxant, antifungal, antibacterial, inhibition of acetylcholinesterase, antiradical, [131–133].	Alkaloids, tannins [132,134].	Myrcene; germacrene D; limonene, β-caryophyllene; decanal [135]. Acide 3,4-O-divanilloylquinique, acide 3,5-O-divanilloylquinique, acide 4,5-O-divanilloylquinique [136].fagaramide; (+)-sésamine; lupéol; hespéridine; Dihydrochélérythrine; N,N-dimethyllindcarpine; Chélérythrine; Norchélérythrine; 6-(2-oxybutyl) dihydrochélérythrine; 6-hydroxy-dihydrochélérythrine; avicine; arnottianamide [131] .
Zizyphus mauritiana Lam.	Antitumor, antibacterial, antioxidant, antimicrobial, anticancer [137,138].	Alkaloids, flavonoids, triterpenoids, tannins, glycoside, phenol, lignin, saponins [137,139].	2H-1-benzopyran-2-one; 9, stigmasterol; stigmastane-3,6-dione [137]. 3-methyl piperidine; o-methyl delta-tochopherol; octacosane; cyclobarbital; squalene; 2,4-dimethyl; thymol TMS; benzoquinoline; γ-sitosterol; hydroprogesterone [138].

Roots (36.2%) and leaves (29%) were the most used organs for the preparation of remedies. These data are in agreement with those observed by Olivier's group [21] and Kantati's group [35]. That would be explained by the availability of these plant parts at all periods in this region, but their effectiveness would be related to the significant accumulation of chemical compounds in these organs [113,140]. However, roots use should lead to some species disappearance. Thus, conservation measures of those are necessary.

Methods of remedies preparation are similar to those observed in other works. The decoction (46.7%) was the most used, followed by the trituration, calcination and aqueous maceration. These results are comparable to those of Zerbo's group works in Sanan's region and Western area of Burkina Faso [16,22], Adetutu's group in the South-western of Nigeria [141] and Kantati's group in Togo [35]. They noted that these methods were the main ones used by traditional healers in these different areas. In phytochemistry, the decoction is considered to be a method allowing complete extraction of bioactive chemical compounds of plants [142]. The aqueous maceration was quoted as being a good method of alkaloids and polyphenols extraction [142,143]. Likewise, the trituration and the calcination methods allow reducing vegetable material to powder or paste, while preserving bioactive molecules. These data could justify the main use of these modes of preparation.

The majority of drugs are administrated orally (drink, 40.8%), the preferential mode of administration in the traditional medicine [67]. However, some are preferentially used by external ways. That would be related to risks that oral use presents for some plants, because of their toxicity or the specificity of the disease [21]. The nasal way is the third most used mode of administration. It has the advantage of allowing a fast access of the active substances in the brain and their best absorption [144].

Results of the ethnobotanical survey corroborate with previous phytochemical studies about traditional uses of plants listed [7,35] and their psychoactive compounds content [69,91]. Indeed, alkaloids are the most known of molecules possessing psychoactive properties [67,145]. Likewise, some flavonoids, steroids and terpenoids were quoted to have psychoactive effect [47,53,146]. These chemical constituents intervene to disturb neurotransmitters activities. They stimulate, inhibit or block liberation, reception or elimination of neurotransmitters [147,148]. Pharmacological results show that the main plants used possess anticonvulsant, anxiolytic, antispasmodic, antinociceptive, analgesic or sedative properties [44,85,111]. This result could confirm the presence of psychoactive compounds in these plants.

5. Conclusions

This study made it possible to report 66 plant species belonging to 51 genera and 32 families used for the treatment of neuropsychiatric diseases. Roots and leaves were the most organs used, the decoction and the trituration were the principal modes of drug preparation. The administration of remedies was done mainly by oral way. Plants identified were quoted to possess psychoactive properties and some chemical contents which could justify that.

Traditional remedies suggested in this study are a real interest in the fight against neuropsychiatric disorders. Then, further researches will be necessary to identify psychoactive compounds from these plants and their acting mechanisms for neuropsychiatric diseases treatment.

Acknowledgments: The authors wish to thank Sidonie Yabré and traditional healers of "Hauts Bassins" region from Burkina Faso for their availability and assistance during survey.

Author Contributions: M.K. and P.Z. conceived and designed the survey; P.T.K. realized the survey; P.T.K. and M.C. analyzed the data; P.T.K. wrote the paper; P.Z. identified the plant specimen; S.G., M.K. and A.C. corrected the manuscript.

Conflicts of Interest: The authors declare no conflict of interest.

References

1. Hele, B.; Metowogo, K.; Mouzou, A.P.; Tossou, R.; Ahounou, J.; Eklu-Gadegbeku, K.; Dansou, P.; Aklikokou, A.K. Enquête ethnobotanique sur les plantes utilisées dans le traitement traditionnel des contusions musculaires au Togo. *Rev. Ivoir. Sci. Technol.* **2014**, *24*, 112–130. (In French).

2. Organisation Mondiale de la Santé (OMS). *Rapport de l'atelier Interrégional de l'OMS sur l'utilisation de la Médecine Traditionnelle dans les soins de santé Primaires*; OMS: Genève, Suisse, 2009. (In French)

3. Organisation Mondiale de la Santé (OMS). *Projet Zéro de Plan D'action Mondial Sur la Santé Mentale 2013–2020*; OMS: Genève, Suisse, 2012. (In French)

4. Yasamy, M.T.; Maulik, P.K.; Tomlinson, M.; Lund, C.; Van Ommeren, M.; Saxena, S. Responsible Governance for Mental Health Research in Low Resource Countries. *PLoS Med.* **2011**, *8*, 1–6. [CrossRef] [PubMed]

5. Fusar-Poli, P.; Deste, G.; Smieskova, R.; Barlati, S.; Yung, A.R.; Howes, O.; Stieglitz, R.-D.; Vita, A.; McGuire, P.; Borgwardt, S. Cognitive Functioning in Prodromal Psychosis: A meta-analysis. *Arch. Gen. Psychiatry* **2012**, *69*, 562–571. [CrossRef] [PubMed]

6. World Health Organization (WHO). *Mental Health Gap Action Programme: Scaling up Care for Mental, Neurological, and Substance Use Disorders*; WHO: Geneva, Switzerland, 2008.

7. Moshi, M.J.; Kagashe, G.A.B.; Mbwambo, Z.H. Plants used to treat epilepsy by Tanzanian traditional healers. *J. Ethnopharmacol.* **2005**, *97*, 327–336. [CrossRef] [PubMed]

8. Diaby, M.A. Etude de la chimie et des activités biologiques de *Daniellia oliveri* (Rolfe, Hutch et Dalz), une plante utilisée dans la prise en charge de l'épilepsie au Mali. Thèse d'Etat, USTT-B, Bamako, Mali, 2014.

9. Starling, J.; Feijo, I. Schizophrénie et autres troubles psychotiques à début précoce. *IACAPAP E-textb. Child Adolesc. Ment. Health* **2012**, 1–24. (In French).

10. Rey-bellet, P. Quoi de neuf dans le traitement des psychoses. *Curr. Opin. Psychiatry* **2015**, 1–26.

11. World Health Organization (WHO). *Regional Strategy for Mental Health 2000–2010*; WHO: Geneva, Switzerland, 2000.

12. Comité Français d'Education pour la Santé (CFES) et MILDT. *Médicaments Psychoactifs*; EURO RSCG: Puteaux, France, 2000. (In French). Available online: http://perso.mediaserv.net/ganja/sarah/sarah/106_fin.pdf (accessed on 8 October 2016).

13. Fouchey, M. Etat des lieux sur l'industrie du médicament. *Rev. Neuropsychol.* **2010**, 1–8. (In French). Available online: http://psychologie-m-fouchey.psyblogs.net/ (accessed on 8 October 2016).

14. Sobiecki, J.F. A preliminary inventory of plants used for psychoactive purposes in southern African healing traditions. *Trans. R. Soc. S. Afr.* **2002**, *57*, 1–24. [CrossRef]

15. Taïwe, G.S.; Kuete, V. Neurotoxicity and Neuroprotective Effects of African Medicinal Plants. In *Toxicological Survey of African Medicinal Plants*; Elsevier: London, UK, 2014; pp. 423–444.

16. Zerbo, P.; Millogo-rasolodimby, J.; Nacoulma-ouedraogo, O.G.; Van Damme, P. Plantes médicinales et pratiques médicales au Burkina Faso: Cas des Sanan. *Bois Forêts des Tropiques* **2011**, *307*, 41–53. (In French).

17. Millogo, H.; Guissou, I.P.; Nacoulma, O.G.; Traoré, A.S. Savoir traditionnel et médicament traditionnels améliorés. In Proceedings of the Colloque: Développement durable et santé dans les pays du sud, le médicament, de la recherche au terrain, Centre Européen de Santé Humanitaire, Lyon, France, Decembre 2005. (In French)

18. Tapsoba, H.; Deschamps, J.-P. Use of medicinal plants for the treatment of oral diseases in Burkina Faso. *J. Ethnopharmacol.* **2006**, *104*, 68–78. [CrossRef] [PubMed]

19. Dakuyo, V. Contribution à l'étude de la pharmacopée traditionnelle burkinabé: Enquête ethnopharmacologique dans la région des Cascades. Ph.D. Thesis, Université de Ouagadougou, Ouagadougou, Burkina Faso, 2010.

20. Nadembega, P.; Boussim, J.I.; Nikiema, J.B.; Poli, F.; Antognoni, F. Medicinal plants in Baskoure, Kourittenga Province, Burkina Faso: An ethnobotanical study. *J. Ethnopharmacol.* **2011**, *133*, 378–395. [CrossRef] [PubMed]

21. Olivier, M.; Zerbo, P.; Boussim, J.I. Les plantes des galeries forestières à usage traditionnel par les tradipraticiens de santé et les chasseurs Dozo Sénoufo du Burkina Faso. *Int. J. Biol. Chem. Sci.* **2012**, *6*, 2170–2191. (In French). [CrossRef]

22. Zerbo, P.; Compaore, M.; Meda, N.T.R.; Lamien-Meda, A.; Kiendrebeogo, M. Potential medicinal plants used by traditional healers in western areas of Burkina Faso. *World J. Pharm. Pharm. Sci.* **2013**, *2*, 6706–6719.

23. Millogo, A.; Kaboré, J.; Preux, P.-M.; Dumas, M. Traitement des adultes épileptiques en milieu hospitalier à Bobo-Dioulasso (Burkina-Faso). *Epilepsies* **2003**, *15*, 37–40. (In French)

24. Traore, M. Etude du profil et de la prise en charge des cas d'abus de drogues dans la ville de Bobo-Bioulasso (Burkina Baso). Ph.D. Thesis, Université de Ouagadougou, Ouagadougou, Burkina Baso, 2012.

25. Millogo, A.; Ratsimbazafy, V.; Nubukpo, P.; Barro, S.; Zongo, I.; Preux, P. Epilepsy and traditional medicine in Bobo-Dioulasso (Burkina Faso). *Acta Neurol. Scand.* **2004**, *109*, 250–254. [CrossRef] [PubMed]

26. Ministère de l'Economie et du Développement (MED). *Profil des Regions du Burkina Faso: La région des Hauts Bassins*; MED: Ouagadougou, Burkina Faso, 2005. (In French)

27. Fontès, J.; Guinko, S. *CARTE de la Végétation et de L'occupation du Sol du Burkina Faso: Notice Explicative*; Université de Toulouse III: Toulouse, France, 1995. (In French)

28. Institut National de la Statistique et de la Démographie (INSD). *Etat et structure de la population*; INSD: Ouagadougou, Burkina Faso, 2009. (In French)

29. Hutchinson, J.; Dalziel, J.M. *Flora of West Tropical Africa*; The Whitefriars Press: Londre/Tonbridge, UK, 1963.

30. Nacoulma-Ouedraogo, O.G. Plantes médicinales et pratiques médicinales traditionnelles au Burkina Faso: Cas du plateau central. Thèse d'Etat, Université de Ouagadougou, Ouagadougou, Burkina Faso, 1996.

31. Thiombiano, A.; Schmidt, M.; Dressler, S.; Ouédraogo, A.; Hahn, K.; Zizka, G. *Catalogue Des Plantes Vasculaires Du BURKINA Faso.* Conservatoire et jardin botaniques de la ville de genève. 2012. Available online: http://www.worldcat.org/title/ (accessed on 8 October 2016).

32. Kerharo, J.; Bouquet, A. *Plantes Médicinales Et Toxiques De La Côte-d'Ivoire-Haute-Volta. Mission D'étude De La Pharmacopée Indigène En A.O.F*; Editions Vigot Frères: Paris, France, 1950. (In French)

33. Pageard, R. Plantes à brûler chez les Bambara. *J. Soc. Afr.* **1967**, *37*, 87–130. [CrossRef]

34. Moreau, R. *Quelques Plantes de Haute-volta: Leurs noms Vernaculaires en Langues Mossi, dioula, bobo-oulé, Dagari et Peul-wassolo*; Publications des scientifiques de l'IRD: Haute-Volta, French, 1970. (In French)

35. Kantati, Y.T.; Kodjo, K.M.; Dogbeavou, K.S.; Vaudry, D.; Leprince, J.; Gbeassor, M. Ethnopharmacological survey of plant species used in folk medicine against central nervous system disorders in Togo. *J. Ethnopharmacol.* **2016**, *181*, 214–220. [CrossRef] [PubMed]

36. Traoré, A.; Derme, A. I.; Sanon, S.; Gansane, A.; Ouattara, Y.; Nebié, I.; Sirima, S.B. Connaissances ethnobotaniques et pratiques phytothérapeutiques des tradipraticiens de santé de la Comoé pour le traitement du paludisme: Processus d'une recherche scientifique de nouveaux antipaludiques au Burkina Faso. *Ethnopharmacologia* **2009**, *43*, 35–46. (In French).

37. Sobiecki, J.F. A review of plants used in divination in southern Africa and their psychoactive effects. *S. Afr. Humanit.* **2008**, *20*, 333–351.

38. Perveen, T.; Haider, S.; Zubairi, N.A.; Ahmed, W.; Batool, Z.; Begum, S. Effect of herbal combination on biochemical and behavioral responses in rats. *Pak. J. Biochem. Mol. Biol.* **2012**, *45*, 20–22.

39. Sucher, N.J.; Carles, M.C. A pharmacological basis of herbal medicines for epilepsy. *Epilepsy Behav.* **2015**, *52*, 308–318. [CrossRef] [PubMed]

40. Bruneton, J. *Pharmacognosie, Phytochimie, Plantes Médicinales*, 2ème ed.; Tec. et Doc.: Lavoisier, Paris, 1993.

41. Sereme, A.; Millogo-Rasolodimby, J.; Guinko, S.; Nacro, M. Proprietes Therapeutiques Des Plantes a Tanins Du Burkina Faso. *Pharmacopée Méd. Tradit. Afr.* **2008**, *15*, 41–49. (In French).

42. Al-snafi, A.E. The constituents and pharmacological properties of Calotropis procera-an overview. *Int. J. Pharm. Rev. Res.* **2015**, *5*, 259–275.

43. Mohamed, N.H.; Liu, M.; Abdel-mageed, W.M.; Alwahibi, L.H.; Dai, H.; Ahmed, M.; Badr, G.; Quinn, R.J.; Liu, X.; Zhang, L.; et al. Cytotoxic cardenolides from the latex of Calotropis procera. *Bioorg. Med. Chem. Lett.* **2015**, *25*, 4615–4620. [CrossRef] [PubMed]

44. Lima, R.C.D.S.; Silva, M.C.C.; Aguiar, C.C.T.; Chaves, E.M.C.; Dias, K.C.F.; Macêdo, D.S.; Sousa, F.C.F.; Carvalho, K.M.; Ramos, M.V.; Mendes, V.M. Anticonvulsant action of Calotropis procera latex proteins. *Epilepsy Behav.* **2012**, *23*, 123–126. [CrossRef] [PubMed]

45. Steenkamp, P.A.; Harding, N.M.; Van Heerden, F.R.; Van Wyk, B.E. Fatal Datura poisoning: Identification of atropine and scopolamine by high performance liquid chromatography/photodiode array/mass spectrometry. *Forensic Sci. Int.* **2004**, *145*, 31–39. [CrossRef] [PubMed]

46. Maiga, A.; Diallo, D.; Fane, S.; Sanogo, R.; Paulsen, B.S.; Cisse, B. A survey of toxic plants on the market in the district of Bamako, Mali: Traditional knowledge compared with a literature search of modern pharmacology and toxicology. *J. Ethnopharmacol.* **2005**, *96*, 183–193. [CrossRef] [PubMed]

47. Zhang, Z. Therapeutic effects of herbal extracts and constituents in animal models of psychiatric disorders. *Life Sci.* **2004**, *75*, 1659–1699. [CrossRef] [PubMed]

48. Marder, M.; Wasowski, C.; Medina, J.H.; Paladini, A.C. 6-Methylapigenin and hesperidin: New valeriana flavonoids with activity on the CNS. *Pharmacol. Biochem. Behav.* **2003**, *75*, 537–545. [CrossRef]
49. Dajas, F.; Rivera, F.; Blasina, F.; Arredondo, F.; Lafon, L.; Morquio, A.; Heizen, H. Cell Culture Protection and in vivo Neuroprotective Capacity of Flavonoids. *Neurotox. Res.* **2003**, *5*, 425–432. [CrossRef] [PubMed]
50. Lake, J. Natural product-derived treatments of neuropsychiatric disorders: Review of progress and recommendations. *Stud. Nat. Prod. Chem.* **2000**, *24*, 1093–1137.
51. Guenne, S.; Balmus, I.M.; Hilou, A.; Ouattara, N.; Kiendrebéogo, M.; Ciobica, A.; Timofte, D. The relevance of Asteraceae family plants in most of the neuropsychiatric disorders treatment. *Int. J. Phyt.* **2016**, *8*, 176–182.
52. Gurib-Fakim, A. Medicinal plants: Traditions of yesterday and drugs of tomorrow. *Mol. Asp. Med.* **2006**, *27*, 1–93. [CrossRef] [PubMed]
53. Becaud-Boyer, A.-S. *Salvia divinorum*, hallucinogène d'aujourd'hui, outil thérapeutique de demain? Thèse d'Etat, Université Joseph FOURIER, Grenoble, France, 2011.
54. Charlene, B. La soumission chimique. Thèse d'Etat, Université Toulouse III, Toulouse, France, 2013.
55. Eldeen, S.; Mohamed, I. Pharmacological investigation of some trees used in South African traditional medicine. Ph.D. Thesis, University of KwaZulu–Natal, Pietermaritzburg, South Africa, 2005.
56. Seigler, D.S.; Butterfield, C.S.; Dunn, J.E.; Conn, E.E. Dihydroacacipetalin–a new cyanogenic glucoside from Acacia sieberiana var. Woodii. *Phytochemistry* **1975**, *14*, 1419–1420. [CrossRef]
57. Salisu, A.; Ogbadu, G.H.; Onyenekwe, P.C.; Olorode, O.; Ndana, R.W.; Segun, O. Evaluating the Nutritional Potential of Acacia Sieberiana Seeds (Dc) Growing in North West of Nigeria. *J. Biol. Life Sci.* **2014**, *5*, 25–36. [CrossRef]
58. Zeuko'o, M.E.; Jurbe, G.G.; Ntim, P.S.; Ajayi, T.A.; Chuwkuka, J.U.; Dawurung, C.J.; Makoshi, M.S.; Elisha, I.L.; Oladipo, O.O.; Lohlum, A.S. Phytochemical Screening and Antidiarrheal Evaluation of Acetone Extract of A cacia sieberiana var woodii (Fabaceae) stem bark in wistar rats. *Acad. J. Pharm. Pharmacol.* **2015**, *3*, 1–6.
59. Uchenna, A.; Nkiruka, V.; Eze, P. Nutrient and Phytochemical Composition of Formulated Diabetic Snacks Made from Two Nigerian Foods Afzelia africana and Detarium microcarpium Seed Flour. *Pak. J. Nutr.* **2013**, *12*, 108–113. [CrossRef]
60. Olajide, O.B.; Fadimu, O.Y.; Osaguona, P.O.; Saliman, M. Botanical and phytochemical studies of some selected species of leguminoseae of northern nigeria: A study of borgu local government area, niger state. Nigeria. *Analysis* **2013**, *4*, 546–551.
61. Igwenyi, I.O.; Azoro, B.N. Proximate and Phytochemical Compositions of Four Indigenous Seeds Used As Soup Thickeners in Ebonyi State Nigeria. *Food Technol.* **2014**, *8*, 35–40.
62. Egwujeh, S.I.; Yusufu, P.A. Chemical compositions of aril cap of African oak (afzelia africana) seed. *J. Food Sci.* **2015**, *3*, 41–47.
63. Gebreyohannes, G.; Gebreyohannes, M. Medicinal values of garlic: A review. *Int. J. Med. Méd. Sci.* **2013**, *5*, 401–408.
64. Bhandari, S.R.; Yoon, M.K.; Kwak, J. Contents of Phytochemical Constituents and Antioxidant Activity of 19 Garlic (Allium sativum L.) Parental Lines and Cultivars. *Hort. Environ. Biotechnol.* **2014**, *55*, 138–147. [CrossRef]
65. Mallet, A.C.T.; Cardoso, M.G.; Souza, P.E.; Machado, S.M.F.; Andrade, M.A.; Nelson, D.L.; Piccoli, R.H. Chemical characterization of the Allium sativum and Origanum vulgare essential oils and their inhibition effect on the growth of some food pathogens. *Rev. Bras. Plant. Med.* **2014**, *16*, 804–811. [CrossRef]
66. Johnson, O.O.; Ayoola, G.A.; Adenipekun, T. Antimicrobial Activity and the Chemical Composition of the Volatile Oil Blend from Allium sativum (Garlic Clove) and Citrus reticulata (Tangerine Fruit). *Int. J. Pharm. Sci. Drug Res.* **2013**, *5*, 187–193.
67. Yinyang, J.; Mpondo, M.E.; Tchatat, M.; Ndjib, R.C.; Mvogo-Ottou, P.B.; Dibong, S.D. Les plantes à alcaloïdes utilisées par les populations de la ville de Douala (Cameroun). *J. Appl. Biosci.* **2014**, *78*, 6600–6619. [CrossRef]
68. Rainy, G.; Amita, S.; Preeti, M. Study of chemical composition of garlic oil and comparative analysis of co-trimoxazole in response to in vitro antibacterial activity. *Int. Res. J. Pharm.* **2014**, *5*, 1–5.
69. Mustapha, A.A. Annona senegalensis Persoon: A Multipurpose shrub, its Phytotherapic, Phytopharmacological and Phytomedicinal Uses. *Int. J. Sci. Technol.* **2013**, *2*, 862–865.

70. Konate, A.; Sawadogo, W.R.; Dubruc, F.; Caillard, O.; Ouedraogo, M. Phytochemical and Anticonvulsant Properties of Annona senegalensis Pers. (Annonaceae), Plant Used in Burkina Folk Medicine to Treat Epilepsy and Convulsions. *Br. J. Pharmacol. Toxicol.* **2012**, *3*, 245–250.

71. Awa, E.P.; Ibrahim, S.; Ameh, D.A. GC/MS Analysis and antimicrobial activity of Diethyl ether fraction of Methanolic extract from the stem bark of Annona senegalensis pers. *Int. J. Pharm. Sci. Res.* **2012**, *3*, 4213–4218.

72. Ibrahim, S.R.M.; Mohamed, G.A.; Shaala, L.A.; Moreno, L.; Banuls, Y.; Van Goietsenoven, G.; Kiss, R.; Youssef, D.T.A. New ursane-type triterpenes from the root bark of Calotropis procera. *Phytochem. Lett.* **2012**, *5*, 490–495. [CrossRef]

73. Patil, S.G.; Patil, M.P.; Maheshwari, V.L.; Patil, R.H. In vitro lipase inhibitory effect and kinetic properties of di-terpenoid fraction from Calotropis procera (Aiton). *Biocatal. Agric. Biotechnol.* **2015**, *4*, 579–585. [CrossRef]

74. Sayed, A.E.H.; Mohamed, N.H.; Ismail, M.A.; Abdel-mageed, W.M.; Shoreit, A.A.M. Antioxidant and antiapoptotic activities of *Calotropis procera* latex on Catfish (Clarias gariepinus) exposed to toxic 4-nonylphenol. *Ecotoxicol. Environ. Saf.* **2016**, *128*, 189–194. [CrossRef] [PubMed]

75. Nenaah, G.E. Potential of using flavonoids, latex and extracts from Calotropis procera (Ait.) as grain protectants against two coleopteran pests of stored rice. *Ind. Crop. Prod.* **2013**, *45*, 327–334. [CrossRef]

76. Kerharo, J.; Adam, J.G. La Pharmacopée sénégalaise traditionnelle. Plantes médicinales et toxiques. ournal d'agriculture Trop. *Bot. Appl.* **1974**, *21*, 76–77.

77. Jeong-Hyun, L.; Jae-Sug, L. Chemical Composition and Antifungal Activity of Plant Essential Oils against Malassezia furfur. *Kor. J. Microbiol. Biotechnol.* **2010**, *38*, 315–321.

78. Dongmo, P.M.J.; Tchoumbougnang, F.; Boyom, F.F.; Sonwa, E.T.; Zollo, P.H.A.; Menut, C. Antiradical, antioxidant activities and anti-inflammatory potential of the essential oils of the varieties of citrus limon and citrus aurantifolia growing in Cameroon. *J. Asian Sci. Res.* **2013**, *3*, 1046–1057.

79. Ouedrhiri, W.; Bouhdid, S.; Balouiri, M.; Lalami, A.E.O.; Moja, S.; Chahdi, F.O.; Greche, H. Chemical composition of Citrus aurantium L. leaves and zest essential oils, their antioxidant, antibacterial single and combined effects. *J. Chem. Pharm. Res.* **2015**, *7*, 78–84.

80. Ahmadu, A.; Haruna, A.K.; Garba, M.; Ehinmidu, J.O.; Sarker, S.D. Phytochemical and antimicrobial activities of the Danieliia oliveri leaves. *Fitoterapia* **2004**, *75*, 729–732. [CrossRef] [PubMed]

81. Kaboré, A. Activité anthelminthique de deux plantes tropicales testée in vitro et in vivo sur les strongles gastro-intestinaux des ovins de race mossi du Burkina Faso. Thèse de Doctorat, Université Polytechnique de Bobo-Dioulasso, Bobo-Dioulasso, Burkina Faso, 2009.

82. Muanda, F.N.; Dicko, A.; Soulimani, R. Assessment of polyphenolic compounds, in vitro antioxydant and anti-inflammation properties of securidaca longepedunculata root barks. *Comptes Rendus Biol.* **2010**, *333*, 663–669. [CrossRef] [PubMed]

83. SOPCFC (Scientific Opinion of the Panel on Contaminants in the Food Chain). Request from the European Commission Tropane alkaloids (from Datura sp.) as undesirable substances in animal feed. *EFSA J.* **2008**, *691*, 1–55.

84. Mahmood, A.; Mahmood, A.; Mahmood, M. In vitro Biological Activities of Most Common Medicinal Plants of Family Solanaceae. *World Appl. Sci. J.* **2012**, *17*, 1026–1032.

85. Maheshwari, N.O.; Khan, A.; Chopade, B.A. Rediscovering the medicinal properties of Datura sp.: A review. *J. Med. Plant. Res.* **2013**, *7*, 2885–2897.

86. Berkov, S.; Zayed, R. Comparison of Tropane Alkaloid Spectra Between *Datura innoxia* Grown in Egypt and Bulgaria. *Z. Naturforsch. C* **2004**, *59*, 184–186. [CrossRef] [PubMed]

87. Lamien-Meda, A.; Lamien, C.E.; Compaoré, M.M.Y.; Meda, R.N.T.; Kiendrebeogo, M.; Zeba, B.; Millogo, J.F.; Nacoulma, O.G. Polyphenol Content and Antioxidant Activity of Fourteen Wild Edible Fruits from Burkina Faso. *Molecules* **2008**, *13*, 581–594. [CrossRef] [PubMed]

88. Belemtougri, R.G.; Constantin, B.; Cognard, C.; Raymond, G.; Sawadogo, L. Effects of two medicinal plants Psidium guajava L. (Myrtaceae) and Diospyros mespiliformis L. (Ebenaceae) leaf extracts on rat skeletal muscle cells in primary culture. *J. Zhejiang Univ. Sci. B* **2006**, *7*, 56–63. [CrossRef] [PubMed]

89. Abdulmalik, I.A.; Sule, M.I.; Musa, A.M.; Yaro, A.H.; Abdullahi, M.I.; Abdulkadir, M.F.; Yusuf, H. Isolation of Steroids from Acetone Extract of Ficus iteophylla. *Br. J. Pharmacol. Toxicol.* **2011**, *2*, 270–272.

90. Soha, P.M.; Benoit-Vical, F. Are West African plants a source of future antimalarial drugs? *J. Ethnopharmacol.* **2007**, *114*, 130–140. [CrossRef] [PubMed]

91. Somboro, A.A.; Patel, K.; Diallo, D.; Sidibe, L.; Chalchat, J.C.; Figueredo, G.; Ducki, S.; Troin, Y.; Chalard, P. An ethnobotanical and phytochemical study of the African medicinal plant *Guiera senegalensis* J. F. Gmel. *J. Med. Plants Res.* **2011**, *5*, 1639–1651.

92. Ouédraogo, F. Etude in vitro de l'activité antiplasmodiale d'extraits de feuilles, de fleurs et de galles de Guiera senegalensis J. F. Gmel (combretaceae). Thèse Doctorat, Université de Ouagadougou, Ouagadougou, Burkina Faso, 2011.

93. Androulakis, X.M.; Muga, S.J.; Chen, F.; Koita, Y.; Toure, B.; Michael Wargovich, J. Chemopreventive Effects of Khaya senegalensis Bark Extract on Human Colorectal Cancer. *Anticancer Res.* **2006**, *26*, 2397–2406. [PubMed]

94. Idu, M.; Igeleke, C.L. Antimicrobial Activity and Phytochemistry of Khaya senegalensis Roots. *Int. J. Ayurvedic Herb. Med.* **2012**, *2*, 415–422.

95. Wakirwa, J.H.; Idris, S.; Madu, S.J.; Dibal, M.; Malgwi, T. Assessment of the In-vitro antimicrobial potential of Khaya Senegalensis ethanol leaf extract. *J. Chem. Pharm. Res.* **2013**, *5*, 182–186.

96. Nwodo, N.J.; Ibezim, A.; Ntie-Kang, F.; Adikwu, M.U.; Mbah, C.J. Anti-Trypanosomal Activity of Nigerian Plants and Their Constituents. *Molecules* **2015**, *2*, 7750–7771. [CrossRef] [PubMed]

97. Atawodi, S.E.; Atawodi, J.C.; Pala, Y.; Idakwo, P. Assessment of the Polyphenol Profile and Antioxidant Properties of Leaves, Stem and Root Barks Of Khaya senegalensis (Desv.) A.Juss. *Electron. J. Biol.* **2009**, *5*, 80–84.

98. Khalid, S.A.; Friedrichsen, G.M.; Kharazmi, A.; Theander, T.G.; Olsen, C.E.; Christensen, S.B. Limonoids from Khaya senegalensis. *Phytochemistry* **1998**, *49*, 1769–1772. [CrossRef]

99. Zongo, C.; Akomo, E.-F.O.; Sawadogo, A.; Obame, L.C.; Koudou, J.; Traore, A.S. In vitro antibacterial properties of total alkaloids extract from Mitragyna inermis (Will) O. Kuntze, a West African traditional medicinal plant. *Asian J. Plant Sci.* **2009**, *8*, 172–177. [CrossRef]

100. Uthman, G.S.; Gana, G.; Zakama, S. Anticonvulsant Screening of the Ethanol Leaf Extract of Mitragyna inermis (Willd) in Mice and Chicks. *Int. J. Res. Pharm. Biomed. Sci.* **2013**, *4*, 1354–1357.

101. Alowanou, G.G.; Olounlade, A.P.; Azando, E.V.B.; Dedehou, V.F.G.N.; Daga, F.D.; Hounzangbeadote, S.M. A review of Bridelia ferruginea, Combretum glutinosum and Mitragina inermis plants used in zootherapeutic remedies in West Africa: Historical origins, current uses and implications for conservation. *J. Appl. Biosci.* **2015**, *87*, 8003–8014. [CrossRef]

102. Konkon, N.G.; Adjoungoua, A.L.; Manda, P.; Simaga, D.; N'Guessan, K.E.; Kone, B.D. Toxicological and phytochemical screening study of Mitragyna Inermis (willd.) O ktze (Rubiaceae), anti-diabetic plant. *J. Med. Plan. Res.* **2008**, *2*, 279–284.

103. Takayama, H.; Ishikawa, H.; Kitajima, M.; Aimi, N.; Aji, B.M. A new 9-methoxyyohimbine-type indole alkaloid from Mitragyna inermis. *Chem. Pharm. Bull.* **2004**, *52*, 359–361. [CrossRef] [PubMed]

104. Cheng, Z.H.; Yua, B.Y.; Yang, X.W. 27-Nor-terpenoid glycosides from Mitragyna inermis. *Phytochemistry* **2002**, *61*, 379–382. [CrossRef]

105. Karou, S.D.; Tchacondo, T.; Ilboudo, D.P.; Simpore, J. Sub-saharan Rubiaceae : A review of their traditional uses, phytochemistry and biological activities. *Pak. J. Biol. Sci.* **2011**, *14*, 149–169. [CrossRef] [PubMed]

106. Ajaiyeoba, E.O. Phytochemical antibacterial properties of parkia biglobosa and parkia bicolor leaf extracts. *Afr. J. Riomed. Res.* **2002**, *5*, 125–129. [CrossRef]

107. Bukar, A.; Uba, A.; Oyeyi, T.I. Phytochemical Analysis and Antimicrobial Activity of Parkia Biglobosa (Jacq.) Benth. Extracts Againt Some Food – Borne Microrganisms. *Adv. Environ. Biol.* **2010**, *4*, 74–79.

108. Komolafe, K.; Akinmoladun, A.C.; Olaleye, M.T. Methanolic leaf extract of Parkia biglobosa protects against doxorubicin-induced cardiotoxicity in rats. *Int. J. Appl. Res. Nat. Prod.* **2013**, *6*, 39–47.

109. Ezekwe, C.I.; Ada, A.C.; Okechukwu, P.C.U. Effects of Methanol Extract of Parkia biglobosa Stem Bark on the Liver and Kidney Functions of Albino Rats. *Glob. J. Biotechnol. Biochem.* **2013**, *8*, 40–50.

110. Adebiyi, R.A.; Elsa, A.T.; Agaie, B.M.; Etuk, E.U. Antinociceptive and antidepressant like effects of Securidaca longepedunculata root extract in mice. *J. Ethnopharmacol.* **2006**, *107*, 234–239. [CrossRef] [PubMed]

111. Adeyemi, O.O.; Akindele, A.J.; Yemitan, O.K.; Aigbe, F.R.; Fagbo, F.I. Anticonvulsant, anxiolytic and sedative activities of the aqueous root extract of Securidaca longepedunculata Fresen. *J. Ethnopharmacol.* **2010**, *130*, 191–195. [CrossRef] [PubMed]

112. Okomolo, C.M.; Mbafor, J.T.; Bum, E.N.; Kouemou, N.; Kandeda, A.K.; Talla, E.; Dimo, T.; Rakotonirira, A.; Rakotonirira, S.V. Evaluation of the sedative and anticonvulsant properties of three Cameroonnian plant. *Afr. J. Tradit. Complement. Altern. Med.* **2011**, *8*, 181–190. [PubMed]

113. Nébié, R.H.C.; Yaméogo, R.T.; Bélanger, A.; Sib, F.S. Salicylate de méthyle, constituant unique de l'huile essentielle de l'écorce des racines de *Securidaca longepedunculata* du Burkina Faso. *C. R. Chim.* **2004**, *7*, 1003–1006. (In French). [CrossRef]

114. Mitaine-offer, A.; Pénez, N.; Miyamoto, T.; Delaude, C.; Mirjolet, J.; Duchamp, O.; Lacaille-dubois, M. Phytochemistry Acylated triterpene saponins from the roots of *Securidaca longepedunculata*. *Phytochemistry* **2010**, *71*, 90–94. [CrossRef] [PubMed]

115. Sow, P.G. Enquête Ethnobotanique et Ethnopharmacologique des Plantes Médicinales de la pharmacopée Sénégalaise Dans le Traitement des Morsures de Serpents. *Le Pharmacien Hospitalier et Clinicien* **2012**, *47*, 37–41. [CrossRef]

116. Van Wyk, B.E.; Van Oudtshoorn, B.; Gericke, N. *Medicinal Plants of South Africa*, 1st ed.; Briza Publications: Pretoria, South Africa, 2005.

117. Diakité, B. La susceptibilite des larves d'Anopheles gambiae S.L. à des extraits de plantes medicinales du Mali. PhD Thesis, Université de Bamako, Bamako, Mali, 2008.

118. Dibwe, D.F.; Awale, S.; Kadota, S.; Morita, H.; Tezuka, Y. Heptaoxygenated xanthones as anti-austerity agents from Securidaca longepedunculata. *Bioorg. Med. Chem.* **2013**, *21*, 7663–7668. [CrossRef] [PubMed]

119. Bhadoriya, S.S.; Mishra, V.; Raut, S.; Ganeshpurkar, A.; Jain, S.K. Anti-Inflammatory and Antinociceptive Activities of a Hydroethanolic Extract of Tamarindus indica Leaves. *Sci. Pharm.* **2012**, *80*, 685–700. [CrossRef] [PubMed]

120. Tariq, M.; Chaudhary, S.; Rahman, K.; Hamiduddin; Zaman, R.; Shaikh, L. Tamarindus indica: An overview. *J. Biol. Sci. Opin.* **2013**, *1*, 128–131. [CrossRef]

121. Yusha'u, M.; Gabari, D.A.; Dabo, N.T.; Hassan, A.; Dahiru, M. Biological activity and phytochemical constituents of Tamarindus indica stem bark extracts. *Sky J. Microbiol. Res.* **2014**, *2*, 67–71.

122. Doughari, J.H. Antimicrobial Activity of Tamarindus indica Linn. *Trop. J. Pharm. Res.* **2006**, *5*, 597–603. [CrossRef]

123. Kapur, M.A.; John, S.A. Antimicrobial Activity of Ethanolic Bark Extract of Tamarindus indica against some Pathogenic Microorganisms. *Int. J. Curr. Microbiol. Appl. Sci.* **2014**, *3*, 589–593.

124. Ahmed, A.O.E.E.; Ayoub, S.M.H. Chemical composition and antimalarial activity of extracts of Sudanese Tamarindus indica L. (Fabaceae). *Pharma Innov. J.* **2015**, *4*, 90–93.

125. Isha, D.; Milind, P. IMLII: A Craze Lovely. *Int. Res. J. Pharm.* **2012**, *3*, 110–115.

126. Maikai, V.A.; Kobo, P.I.; Maikai, B.V.O. Antioxidant properties of Ximenia Americana. *Afr. J. Biotechnol.* **2010**, *9*, 7744–7746.

127. Monte, F.J.Q.; de Lemos, T.L.G.; de Araújo, M.R.S.; Gomes, E.S. Ximenia americana: Chemistry, Pharmacology and Biological Properties, a Review. 2012. Available online: www.intechopen.com (accessed on 12 December 2016).

128. Araújo, M.R.S.; Assunção, J.C.C.; Dantas, I.N.F.; Costa-Lotufo, L.V.; Monte, F.J.Q. Chemical Constituents of Ximenia americana. *Nat.Prod. Commun.* **2008**, *3*, 857–860.

129. Fatope, M.O.; Adoum, O.A.; Takeda, Y. C18 Acetylenic Fatty Acids of Ximenia americana with Potential Pesticidal Activity. *J. Agric. Food Chem.* **2000**, *4*, 1872–1874. [CrossRef]

130. Saeed, A.E.M.; Bashier, R.S.M. Physico-chemical analysis of Ximenia americana L. oil and structure elucidation of some chemical constituents of its seed oil and fruit pulp. *J. Pharmacogn. Phytother.* **2010**, *2*, 49–55.

131. Kouri, F.C. Investigation phytochimique d'une brosse à dents africaine Zanthoxylum zanthoxyloides (Lam.) Zepernick et Timler (Syn. Fagara zanthoxyloides L.) (Rutaceae). Thèse, Université de Lausanne, Lausanne, Suisse, 2004.

132. Gansane, A.; Sanon, S.; Ouattara, P.L.; Hutter, S.; Olivier, E.; Azas, N.; Traore, A.S.; Guissou, I.P.; Nebie, I.; Sirima, B.S. Antiplasmodial activity and cytotoxicity of semi purified fraction: Zanthoxylum zanthoxyloïdes Lam. Bark of trunk. *Int. J. Pharm.* **2010**, *6*, 921–925. [CrossRef]

133. Ouedraogo, S.; Traore, A.; Lompo, M.; Some, N.; Sana, B.; Guissou, I.P. Vasodilator effect of Zanthoxylum zanthoxyloïdes, Calotropis procera and FACA, a mixture of these two plants. *Int. J. Biol. Chem. Sci.* **2011**, *5*, 1351–1357. [CrossRef]

134. Olounladé, P.A.; Hounzangbé-Adoté, M.S.; Azando, E.V.B.; TAmha, T.B.; Brunet, S.; Moulis, C.; Fabre, N.; Fouraste, I.; Hoste, H.; Valentin, A. Etude in vitro de l'effet des tanins de Newbouldia laevis et de Zanthoxylum zanthoxyloïdes sur la migration des larves infestantes de Haemonchus contortus. *Int. J. Biol. Chem. Sci.* **2011**, *5*, 1414–1422.

135. Affouet, K.M.; Tonzibo, Z.F.; Attioua, B.K.; Chalchat, J.C. Chemical Investigations of Volatile Oils from Aromatic Plants Growing in Côte d'ivoire: *Harisonia abyssinica* Oliv., *Canarium schwerfurthii* Engl. *Zanthoxylum gilletti* (De wild) Waterm. And *Zanthoxylum zanthoxyloides* Lam. *Anal. Chem. Lett.* **2012**, *2*, 367–372.

136. Ouattara, B.; Angenot, L.; Guissou, P.; Fondu, P.; Dubois, J.; Frédérich, M.; Jansen, O.; Van Heugen, J.C.; Wauters, J.N.; Tits, M. LC/MS/NMR analysis of isomeric divanilloylquinic acids from the root bark of Fagara zanthoxyloides Lam. *Phytochemistry* **2004**, *65*, 1145–1151. [CrossRef] [PubMed]

137. Sameera, N.S.; Mandakini, B.P. Investigations into the antibacterial activity of Ziziphus mauritiana Lam. and Ziziphus xylopyra (Retz.) Willd. *Int. Food Res. J.* **2015**, *22*, 849–853.

138. Ashraf, A.; Sarfraz, R.A.; Anwar, F.; Shahid, S.A.; Alkharfy, K.M. Chemical composition and biological activities of leaves of Ziziphus mauritiana l. Native to Pakistan. *Pak. J. Bot.* **2015**, *47*, 367–376.

139. Parmar, P.; Bhatt, S.; Dhyani, D.S.; Jain, A. Phytochemical studies of the secondary metabolites of Ziziphus mauritiana Lam. Leaves. *Int. J. Curr. Pharm. Res.* **2012**, *4*, 153–155.

140. Springer, T.L.; Mcgraw, R.L.; Aiken, G.E.; Michx, L. Variation of Condensed Tannins in Roundhead Lespedeza Germplasm. *Crop Sci.* **2002**, *42*, 2157–2160. [CrossRef]

141. Adetutu, A.; Morgan, W.A.; Corcoran, O. Ethnopharmacological survey and in vitro evaluation of wound-healing plants used in South-western Nigeria. *J. Ethnopharmacol.* **2011**, *137*, 50–56. [CrossRef] [PubMed]

142. Kalla, A. Etude et valorisation des principes actifs de quelques plantes du sud algérien: *Pituranthos scoparius, Rantherium adpressum* et *Traganum nudatum*. Ph.D. Thesis, Université Mentouri-Constantine, Constantine, Algérie, 2012.

143. Feknous, S.; Saidi, F.; Said, R.M. Extraction, caractérisation et identification de quelques métabolites secondaires actifs de la mélisse (*Melissa officinalis* L.). *Nat. Technol.* **2014**, *11*, 7–13.

144. Mohagheghzadeh, A.; Faridi, P.; Shams-ardakani, M.; Ghasemi, Y. Medicinal smokes. *J. Ethnopharmacol.* **2006**, *108*, 161–184. [CrossRef] [PubMed]

145. Ujváry, I. Psychoactive natural products: Overview of recent developments. *Ann Ist Super Sanità* **2014**, *50*, 12–27. [PubMed]

146. Amar, B.M. *La Polyconsommation de Psychotropes et les Principales Interactions Pharmacologiques Associées*; Centre québécois de lutte aux dépendances: Québec, QC, Canada, 2007.

147. Organisation Mondiale de la Santé (OMS). *Neurosciences: Usage de Substances Psychoactives et Dépendance*; OMS: Genève, Suisse, 2004.

148. Stafford, G.I.; Jäger, A.K.; Van Staden, J. African Psychoactive Plants. *Challenges* **2009**, *1021*, 323–346.

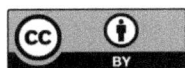

medicines

MDPI

Article

Compounds from *Terminalia mantaly* L. (Combretaceae) Stem Bark Exhibit Potent Inhibition against Some Pathogenic Yeasts and Enzymes of Metabolic Significance

Marthe Aimée Tchuente Tchuenmogne [1], Thierry Ngouana Kammalac [2], Sebastian Gohlke [3], Rufin Marie Toghueo Kouipou [2], Abdulselam Aslan [4], Muslum Kuzu [5], Veysel Comakli [6], Ramazan Demirdag [6], Silvère Augustin Ngouela [1], Etienne Tsamo [1], Norbert Sewald [3], Bruno Ndjakou Lenta [7,*] and Fabrice Fekam Boyom [2,*]

[1] Laboratory of Natural Products and Organic Synthesis, Department of Organic Chemistry, Faculty of Science, University of Yaoundé 1, P.O. Box 812, Yaoundé, Cameroon; tch_aimee@yahoo.fr (M.A.T.T.); sngouela@yahoo.fr (S.A.N.); tsamoet@yahoo.fr (E.T.)
[2] Antimicrobial & Biocontrol Agents Unit, Laboratory for Phytobiochemistry and Medicinal Plants Studies, Department of Biochemistry, Faculty of Science, University of Yaoundé I, P.O. Box 812, Yaoundé, Cameroon; ngouanathi@yahoo.com (T.N.K.); toghueo.rufin@yahoo.fr (R.M.T.K.)
[3] Chemistry Department, Organic and Bioorganic Chemistry, Bielefeld University, P.O. Box 100131, D-33501 Bielefeld, Germany; sebastian.gohlke@uni-bielefeld.de (S.G.); norbert.sewald@uni-bielefeld.de (N.S.)
[4] Faculty of Engineering, Department of Industrial Engineering, Giresun University, 28200 Giresun, Turkey; abdulselam@hotmail.de
[5] Faculty of Pharmacy, Department of Basic Pharmaceutical Sciences, Agrı Ibrahim Cecen University, 04100 Agri, Turkey; mkuzu@agri.edu.tr
[6] School of Health, Department of Nutrition and Dietetics, Agrı Ibrahim Cecen University, 04100 Agri, Turkey; veysel_comakli@hotmail.com (V.C.); r.demirdag@hotmail.com (R.D.)
[7] Department of Chemistry, Higher Teacher Training College, University of Yaoundé 1, Yaoundé, Cameroon
* Correspondence: lentabruno@yahoo.fr (B.N.L.); fabrice.boyom@fulbrightmail.org (F.F.B.); Tel.: +237-675-097-561 (B.N.L.); +237-677-276-585 (F.F.B.)

Academic Editor: James D. Adams
Received: 1 November 2016; Accepted: 12 January 2017; Published: 24 January 2017

Abstract: Background: Pathogenic yeasts resistance to current drugs emphasizes the need for new, safe, and cost-effective drugs. Also, new inhibitors are needed to control the effects of enzymes that are implicated in metabolic dysfunctions such as cancer, obesity, and epilepsy. **Methods:** The anti-yeast extract from *Terminalia mantaly* (Combretaceae) was fractionated and the structures of the isolated compounds established by means of spectroscopic analysis and comparison with literature data. Activity was assessed against *Candida albicans*, *C. parapsilosis* and *C. krusei* using the microdilution method, and against four enzymes of metabolic significance: glucose-6-phosphate dehydrogenase, human erythrocyte carbonic anhydrase I and II, and glutathione *S*-transferase. **Results:** Seven compounds, 3,3′-di-*O*-methylellagic acid 4′-*O*-α-rhamnopyranoside; 3-*O*-methylellagic acid; arjungenin or 2,3,19,23-tetrahydroxyolean-12-en-28-oïc acid; arjunglucoside or 2,3,19,23-tetrahydroxyolean-12-en-28-oïc acid glucopyranoside; 2α,3α,24-trihydroxyolean-11,13(18)-dien-28-oïc acid; stigmasterol; and stigmasterol 3-*O*-β-d-glucopyranoside were isolated from the extract. Among those, 3,3′-di-*O*-methylellagic acid 4′-*O*-α-rhamnopyranoside, 3-*O*-methylellagic acid, and arjunglucoside showed anti-yeast activity comparable to that of reference fluconazole with minimal inhibitory concentrations (MIC) below 32 μg/mL. Besides, Arjunglucoside potently inhibited the tested enzymes with 50% inhibitory concentrations (IC$_{50}$) below 4 μM and inhibitory constant (Ki) <3 μM. **Conclusions:** The results achieved indicate that further SAR studies will likely identify potent hit derivatives that should subsequently enter the drug development pipeline.

Keywords: *Terminalia mantaly*; Combretaceae; anti-yeast; enzyme inhibitors

---

1. Introduction

Fungal diseases affect 3–4 million people worldwide every year. Of particular importance, the increasing resistance of pathogenic opportunistic yeasts to current drugs is a serious concern and has attracted the attention of the scientific community. New, safe, and cost-effective drugs of natural or synthetic origin are therefore actively being researched [1]. Recent epidemiological data highlight the increasing burden of pathogenic yeasts on people in poor settings [2–4]. *Candida* species and *Cryptococcus neoformans* are the major pathogenic yeasts and only a few antifungal drugs have been developed so far to treat the invasive infections they cause [5,6]. Medicinal plants have shown credibility as sources of treatment for infectious diseases [7]. In Cameroon, extracts from medicinal plants such as *Terminalia mantaly* (Combretaceae) are widely used by traditional healers to control diverse infections or associated symptoms, including but not limited to dysentery, gastroenteritis, hypertension, diabetes, and oral, dental, cutaneous and genital affections [8]. Previous studies on the extracts of this plant have showed antibacterial and antifungal properties, but their chemical compositions have not yet been determined [9]. However, phytochemical studies of other species of the genus *Terminalia* have reported the presence of flavonoids, terpenoids and their glycosides derivatives, tannins, flavonones and chalcones [10–18]. In spite of the work done on *Terminalia* species, no investigation has been attempted yet on the enzyme inhibition properties of their extracts and constituents targeting glucose-6-phosphate dehydrogenase, carbonic anhydrase and glutathione *S*-transferase.

Glucose-6-phosphate dehydrogenase (G6PD; EC 1.1.1.49) is an enzyme that catalyzes the reaction of glucose-6-phosphate into phosphogluconate, which is the rate-limiting first step of the pentose phosphate pathway. The end products of this pathway are ribose-5-phosphate and NADPH. Ribose-5-phosphate is used in DNA or RNA synthesis in cell reproduction, and NADPH is used as a coenzyme for the enzymes participating in the production of reduced glutathione. Given its role in cell growth, this enzyme is of high importance to mammal cells [19,20]. However, several studies have shown that this enzyme has an important role in the pathology of some diseases like cancer, hypertension, heart failure and type 2 diabetes. G6PD activity increases in cancer cells and its inhibition results in decreased cell proliferation and induction of apoptosis. For example, 6-aminonicotinamide, which is an inhibitor of G6PD, has found use in the therapy of various tumors in the past [21].

The carbonic anhydrase (CA; carbonate hydro-lyase, EC 4.2.1.1) enzyme exists commonly in living organisms, and has various isoenzymes according to conditions and necessities of the medium. It is one of the most studied enzymes and CAI and CAII are the most common isoenzymes [22]. In many physiological and pathological processes, CAs catalyze the conversion of CO_2 to HCO_3^- and H^+. In addition, CA inhibitors may be used in the treatment of various diseases such as oedema, glaucoma, obesity, cancer, epilepsy and osteoporosis [23].

In living cells, the deleterious effects of free radicals and their intermediates are eliminated or minimized by various enzymatic and non-enzymatic defense systems. Enzymatic defense is provided by several enzymes such as glutathione *S*-transferase (GST), glutathione reductase, glutathione peroxidase, superoxide dismutase, and catalase [24]. The GSTs (EC 2.5.1.18) are a group of multifunctional enzymes that play an important role in animal metabolism [25]. GSTs are important for the fight against cancer because of their interactions with carcinogens and chemotherapeutic agents. They are the target of antiasthmatic and antitumor drugs [26]. Production of excessive amounts of GST in mammalian tumor cells leads to resistance to some anticancer drugs and chemical carcinogens [27].

The reduction of drug effects in tumor cells is an important factor limiting the therapeutic efficacy of an antineoplastic agent. Over time, the development of this resistance is associated with glutathione (GSH) and glutathione *S*-transferase (GST) levels in cells and changes in permeability to the drug. In this regard, G6PD, CA I, II or GST inhibitors may be useful because of their several applications, in particular for the treatment of glaucoma, epilepsy, cancer and as diuretics.

In our search for bioactive secondary metabolites from Cameroonian medicinal plants, we have investigated the MeOH extract of the stem bark of *T. mantaly* L. (Combretaceae) that previously showed anti-yeast activity. We report in this paper the inhibitory potential of compounds isolated from this extract against some pathogenic yeasts and some enzymes of metabolic significance.

2. Materials and Methods

2.1. General Experimental Procedures

The physicochemical analyses of the isolated natural products were essentially performed as previously described [28]. Optical rotations were measured on a JASCO digital polarimeter (model DIP-3600, JASCO, Tokyo, Japan). UV spectra were determined on a Spectronic Unicam spectrophotometer (Thermo Scientific, Waltham, MA, USA). IR spectra were determined on a JASCO Fourier transform IR-420 spectrometer (JASCO, Tokyo, Japan). ^{1}H and ^{13}C NMR spectra were run on a Bruker spectrometer (Bruker Corporation, Brussels, Belgium) equipped with 5 mm ^{1}H and ^{13}C probes operating at 500 and 125 MHz, respectively, with Tetramethylsilane (TMS) as internal standard. Silica gel 230–400 mesh (Merck, Bielefeld, Germany) and silica gel 70–230 mesh (Merck) were used for flash and column chromatography while precoated aluminum-backed silica gel 60 F254 sheets were used for TLC. Spots were visualized under UV light (254 and 365 nm) or using MeOH–H$_2$SO$_4$ reagent.

2.2. Plant Material

The stem bark of *T. mantaly* (Combretaceae) was collected in Yaoundé, Cameroon in May 2012 and identified at the Cameroon National Herbarium where a voucher specimen is deposited under the reference N° 64212/HNC (*T. mantaly* H. Perrier).

2.3. Microbial Isolates

Yeast isolates were kindly provided by the Laboratory of Clinical Biology, Yaoundé Central Hospital and consisted of clinical isolates of *C. albicans*, *C. krusei* and *C. parapsilosis*. Yeasts were maintained at room temperature and cultured at 37 °C for 24 h on Sabouraud Dextrose Agar (Oxoid, Drongen, Belgium) slants prior to use.

2.4. Plant Extraction and Screening of Anti-Yeast Activity

The harvested *T. mantaly* stem bark was dried at room temperature and ground using a blender. The powdered stem bark (7 kg) was extracted at r.t. with MeOH (48 h). The extract was concentrated under vacuum to afford a dark residue (250 g). Minimal inhibitory concentration (MIC) of the extract was determined according to the CLSI M27-A3 [6] protocol with little modifications. The RPMI 1640 supplemented with 2% glucose was used as culture medium. Briefly for the fungal susceptibility tests, 50 µL of serially two-fold diluted concentrations of the crude extract were added in triplicate wells of a 96-wells microtiter plate. Fifty µL of fungal inocula standardized to a final concentration of 0.5–2.5 × 10^3 CFU/mL were then individually added in each well of the plate. Plant crude extract and the positive control (fluconazole) at concentrations of 0.12 to 64 µg/mL were tested in a final volume of 100 µL. So-prepared plates were incubated at 37 °C for 48 h. MIC value was subsequently determined through macroscopic observation of plate wells, and was defined as the lowest concentration of the inhibitor that allowed no visible growth of the microorganism after overnight incubation compared to the growth control.

2.5. Isolation of Compounds and Screening for Activity

A portion of 180 g of the extract was subjected to medium pressure flash chromatography over silica gel (Merck, 70–230 mesh) using mixtures *n*-hexane-EtOAc of increasing polarity ((70:30)–(0:100)) and EtOAc–MeOH ((95:5)–(50:50)), resulting in the collection of 75 fractions of 500 mL each, which were combined on the basis of TLC analysis to create four fractions labeled T_1–T_4. Fraction T_1 (m = 14.4 g) obtained from the mixtures of *n*-hexane-EtOAc (100:0 to 70:30) was subjected to silica gel column chromatography, eluted with *n*-hexane-EtOAc, and yielded oils stigmasterol (23 mg) and arjungenin (7 mg). From fraction T_2 (m = 60.3 g), eluted with *n*-hexane-EtOAc ((50:50)–(25:75)), stigmasterol 3-*O*-β-D-glucopyranoside (12 mg), arjungenin (17 mg), 2α,3α,24-trihydroxyolean-11,13(18)-dien-28-oic acid (5.0 mg) and arjunglucoside (6 mg) were isolated. Column chromatography of fraction T_3 (m = 55.0 g) on silica gel and eluted with the mixtures of EtOAc–MeOH ((100:0)–(85:15)), yielded 3,3′-di-*O*-methylellagic acid 4′-*O*-α-rhamnopyranoside (32 mg), arjungenin (12.0 mg), arjunglucoside (3.5 mg), 2α,3α,24-trihydroxyolean-11,13(18)-dien-28-oic acid (3.5 mg) and a dark mixture that was subjected to column chromatography on Sephadex LH-20 with MeOH as an isocratic eluent and yielded 3-*O*-methyl ellagic acid (12.5 mg). Fraction T_4 (m = 56.18 g) obtained with the solvent system of EtOAc–MeOH (85:15 to 65:35) was a complex mixture and thus was not studied. All the isolated compounds were screened as described above for anti-yeast activity, and as described below for enzyme inhibition activities.

2.6. Purification of Glucose 6-Phosphate Dehydrogenase and Activity Determination

G6PD was purified from the gill tissue of Lake Van fish according to Kuzu et al. [29], and the enzyme activity was determined spectrophotometrically using a Shimadzu UV-1800 spectrophotometer (Shimadzu, Tokyo, Japan) at 25 °C, according to the method described by Beutler [30] and based on the principle of the reduction of NADP$^+$ to NADPH in the presence of glucose 6-phosphate and absorbance recorded at 340 nm.

2.7. Purification of Carbonic Anhydrase Isoenzymes by Affinity Chromatography and Activity Determination

The purification of hCA I and II isozymes was performed with a simple one step method by a Sepharose-4B anilinesulphanilamide affinity column chromatograph as previously described [31]. Briefly, CNBr activated Sepharose-4B was washed with ddH$_2$O and tyrosine further attached to the activated gel as a spacer arm and finally diazotized sulphanilamide clamped with tyrosine molecule as ligand. The homogenate was applied to the prepared Sepharose-4B-L-Tyrosine Sulphanilamide affinity column equilibrated with 25 mM Tris–HCl/0.1 M Na$_2$SO4 (pH 8.7) (Sigma-Aldrich, Taufkirchen, Germany). The affinity gel was washed with 25 mM Tris–HCl/22 mM Na$_2$SO4 (pH 8.7).

The esterase activity was assessed following the change in absorbance of 4-nitrophenylacetate (NPA) to 4-nitrophenylate ion at 348 nm over a period of 3 min at 25 °C using a Beckman Coulter UV-VIS spectrophotometer (Beckman Coulter, Atlanta, GA, USA) according to the method described by Verpoorte et al. [32].

2.8. Purification of Glutathione S-Transferase Enzyme and Activity Determination

Firstly, heamolysate from human erythrocytes was prepared according to the method of Hunaiti et al. [33]. The prepared heamolysate was directly applied to the glutathione-agarose affinity column and washed with 10 mM KH$_2$PO$_4$ and 0.1 M KCl (pH 8.0) (Sigma-Aldrich). The washing procedure was monitored on a spectrophotometer through equal–to–blind absorbance values. After the column was stabilized, the enzyme was purified by gradient elution at +4 °C [24,34]. Elution solvent was prepared from a solvent gradient containing 50 mM Tris–HCl and (1.25–10 mM GSH, pH 9.5). Thereafter, 1-chloro-2,4-dinitrobenzene (Sigma-Aldrich) was used to determine GST enzyme activity. In fact the complex obtained using dinitrobenzene S-glutathione (DNB-SG) displays maximum absorbance at 340 nm. Activity measurements were thus carried out using the absorbance increment at this wavelength. [35].

2.9. In Vitro Inhibition and Kinetic Studies

To determine the effects of compounds on enzymes, enzyme activities were measured with saturated substrate concentration and five different inhibitor concentrations. The 50% inhibitory concentrations (IC_{50}) were determined by plotting curves of percent inhibition versus compound concentration. Results are reported as IC_{50} values. Ki constants were calculated using the Cheng-Prusoff equation [36].

3. Results and Discussion

The methanol extract of the stem bark of *T. mantaly* was screened for anti-yeast activity in vitro against three clinical isolates consisting of *C. albicans*, *C. krusei* and *C. parapsilosis*. The crude extract exhibited good activity with MIC values of 24 µg/mL against *C. parapsilosis* and 39 µg/mL against *C. albicans* and *C. krusei* (Table 1).

Table 1. Anti-yeast activity of *Terminalia mantaly* extract and isolates.

Extract/Fractions		*C. parapsilosis*	*C. albicans*	*C. krusei*
		MIC * (µg/Ml ± SD)		
MeOH Extract		24.00 ± 0.21	39.00 ± 0.33	39.00 ± 0.30
Fraction T1		1250.00 ± 1.23	2500.00 ± 0.98	2500.00 ± 1.03
Fraction T2		39.00 ± 0.38	>5000	>5000
Fraction T3		0.16 ± 0.02	0.64 ± 0.12	0.02 ± 0.09
Fraction T4		>5000	>5000	>5000
Fraction of origin				
3,3′-di-O-methylellagic acid 4′-O-α-rhamnopyranoside	T3	39.00 ± 0.88 (80.4 µM)	9.70 ± 0.72 (20 µM)	>5000 (10,300 µM)
3-O-methyl ellagic acid	T3	78.00 ± 0.92 (247.6 µM)	156.00 ± 1.00 (495 µM)	19.50 ± 0.57 (61.9 µM)
Arjungenin	T1, T2, T3	>5000 (9487 µM)	>5000 (9487 µM)	>5000 (9487 µM)
Arjunglucoside	T2, T3	39.00 ± 0.13 (56.60 µM)	9.70 ± 0.36 (14.07 µM)	312.00 ± 1.04 (452 µM)
2α,3α,24-trihydroxyolean-11, 13(18)-dien-28-oic acid	T1, T3	>5000 (9823 µM)	>5000 (9823 µM)	>5000 (9823 µM)
Fluconazole **		2.00 ± 0.01 (6.53 µM)	8.00 ± 0.25 (26.14 µM)	32.00 ± 0.42 (10.45 µM)

* Plant extracts were tested using the CLSI M27-A3 protocol. Activity was expressed as minimal inhibitory concentration; ** Reference used as positive control. MIC, minimum inhibitory concentration.

The flash chromatography of the crude extract generated four fractions exhibiting varying antifungal activities. As shown in Table 1, fraction T3 was the most active, with activity magnification over 1950 times against *C. krusei* (MIC = 0.02 µg/mL), 150 times against *C. parapsilosis* (MIC = 0.16 µg/mL), and over 60 times against *C. albicans* (0.64 µg/mL), compared to the crude extract (MIC = 24–39 µg/mL). *C. krusei* was the most susceptible isolate to fraction T3. Compounds 3,3′-di-O-methylellagic acid-4′-O-α-rhamnopyranoside, 3-O-methylellagic acid, arjungenin, arjunglucoside, and 2α,3α,24-trihydroxyolean-11,13(18)-dien-28-oic acid that were all found in fraction T3 were also tested for biological activity (Table 1; Figure 1). Overall, they showed drastically reduced potency against the tested yeasts compared to the mother fraction T3, indicating that fractionation has negatively affected the biological activity. Compounds stigmasterol and stigmasterol 3-*O*-β-D-glucopyranoside were not tested due to reduced solubility in the culture medium. Among the tested compounds, 3,3'-di-*O*-methylellagic acid-4'-*O*-α-rhamnopyranoside and arjunglucoside showed the best potency against *C. albicans* with an MIC of 9.7 µg/mL. They also moderately inhibited *C. parapsilosis* with an MIC of 39 µg/mL. In addition, compound 3-*O*-methylellagic acid inhibited *C. krusei* with an MIC of 19.5 µg/mL.

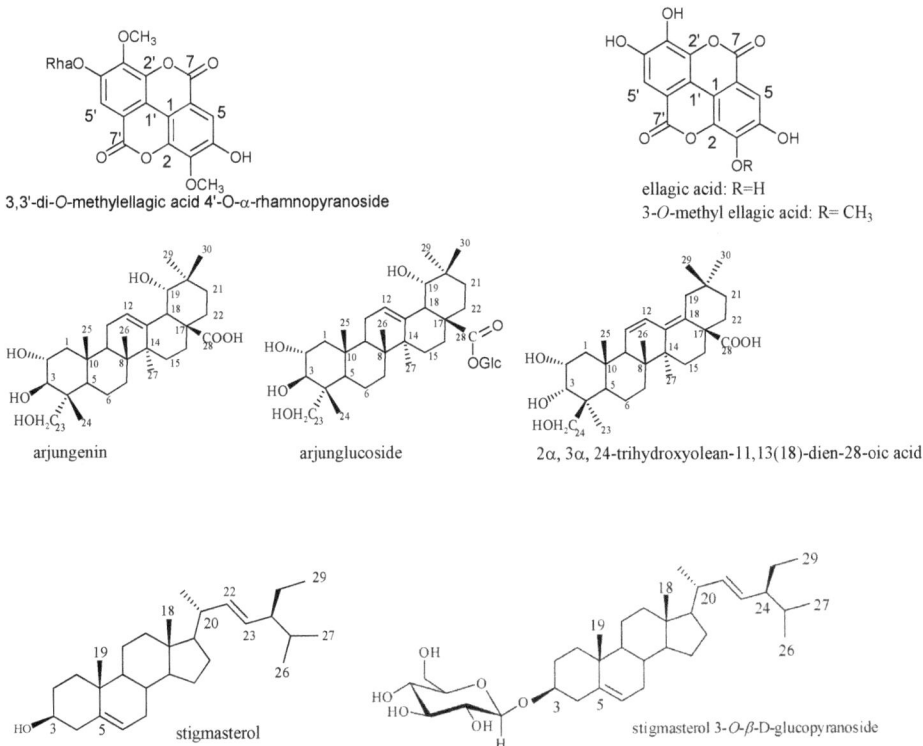

Figure 1. Structures of the isolated compounds from *Terminalia mantaly* (Combretaceae). The isolated compounds were tested against pathogenic yeast isolates and enzymes of metabolic significance. 3,3'-di-*O*-methylellagic acid 4'-*O*-α-rhamnopyranoside: IC_{50} = 39 µg/mL *C. parapsilosis*; 9.7 µg/mL *C. albicans*; >5000 µg/mL *C. krusei*; CAI: IC_{50} = 53.31 µM, Ki = 44.11 µM; CAII: IC_{50} = 69.11 µM, Ki = 55.78 µM; GST: IC_{50} = 63.01 µM, Ki = 42.00 µM. 3-*O*-methyl ellagic acid: IC_{50} = 78 µg/mL *C. parapsilosis*; 156 µg/mL *C. albicans*; 19.5 µg/mL *C. krusei*. arjungenin: *C. parapsilosis*, *C. albicans*, *krusei*: IC_{50} > 5000 µg/mL; CAI: IC_{50} = 86.64 µM, Ki = 71.68 µM; GST: IC_{50} = 1.51 µM, Ki = 1.00 µM; arjunglucoside: IC_{50} = 39 µg/mL *C. parapsilosis*; 9.7 µg/mL *C. albicans*; 312 µg/mL *C. krusei*; G6PD: IC_{50} = 1.84 µM, Ki = 0.19 µM; CAI: IC_{50} = 3.28 µM, Ki = 2.72 µM; CAII: IC_{50} = 1.28 µM, Ki = 1.03 µM; GST: IC_{50} = 1.84 µM, Ki = 1.23 µM. 2α,3α,24-trihydroxyolean-11,13(18)-dien-28-oic acid: IC_{50} > 5000 µg/mL *C. parapsilosis*, *C. albicans*, *C. krusei*.

4. NMR Spectral Data of the Tested Compounds

The physicochemical profiles of the isolated compounds were acquired following previously described approaches [37–40].

3,3′-di-O-methylellagic acid 4′-O-α-rhamnopyranoside. Yellowish powder; molecular formula $C_{21}H_{18}O_{12}$; ESI-MS: [M + Na]$^+$ *m/z* 485,049 ^{1}H-NMR (300 MHz, DMSO-d_6): δ_H 1.13 (3 H, d, CH$_3$, H-6″), 3.54 (1 H, q, *J* = 8.0 and 12.0 Hz, H-5″), 4.01 (1 H, t, H-4″), 4.04 (3 H, s, OMe-3), 4.72 (1 H, brd, *J* = 8.0 Hz, H-3″), 4.94 (1 H, brd, *J* = 4.0 Hz, H-2″), 5.47 (1 H, brs, H-1″), 7.52 (1 H, s, H-5), 7.73 (1 H, s, H-5′); ^{13}C-NMR (125 MHz, DMSO-d_6), aglycone moiety: δ_C 113.4 (C-1), 140.5 (C-2), 141.8 (C-3), 153.1 (C-4), 111.9 (C-5), 113.4 (C-6), 159.1 (C-7), 114.7 (C-1′), 136.6 (C-2′), 142.2 (C-3′), 146.9 (C-4′), 112.0 (C-5′), 107.4 (C-6′), 159.1 (C-7′); rhamnose moiety: 100.5 (C-1″), 70.4 (C-2″), 70.5 (C-3″), 72.2 (C-4″), 70.3 (C-5″), 18.3 (C-6″) and 61.4 (C-3, OMe).

3-O-methyl ellagic acid. Yellowish powder; molecular formula $C_{15}H_8O_8$; ESI-MS: [M − H]$^-$ *m/z* 315, ^{1}H-NMR (DMSO-d_6): δ 7.50 (1 H, s, H-5), 7.44 (1 H, s, H-5′), 4.02 (3 H, s, 3-OMe). ^{13}C-NMR (DMSO-d_6): δ 158.9 (C-7), 158.6 (C-7′), 152.2 (C-4), 148.2 (C-4′), 141.7 (C-2), 140.0 (C-3), 139.8 (C-3′), 136.1 (C-2′), 112.4(C-1′), 112.1 (C-6), 111.7 (C-1), 111.3 (C-5), 110.1 (C-5′), 107.2 (C-6′), 60.8 (3-OMe).

Arjungenin or 2,3,19,23-tetrahydroxyolean-12-en-28-oic acid. White powder; molecular formula $C_{30}H_{48}O_6$; ESI-MS: [M + Na]$^+$ *m/z* 527,322. ^{1}H-NMR (300 MHz, DMSO-d_6): δ_H 1.23, 1.09, 0.90, 0.88, 0.84 and 0.65 (each 3 H, s); 2.92 (1 H, brs, H-18); 2.86 (1 H, d, *J* = 8 Hz, H-3) and 3.57 (1 H, m, H-2); 5.23 (1 H, brs, H-12); ^{13}C-NMR (125 MHz; DMSO-d_6): δ_C 16.8, 17.1, 23.9, 24.9, 28.9 and 24.5; 64.3 (C-23), 80.5 (C-3), 179.6 (C-28), 122.6 (C-12); 143.9 (C-13).

Arjunglucoside or 2,3,19,23-tetrahydroxyolean-12-en-28-oïc acid glucopyranoside. White powder; molecular formula $C_{36}H_{58}O_{11}$; ESI-MS: [M + Na]$^+$ *m/z* 689,396; ^{1}H-NMR (300 MHz, DMSO-d_6): δ 1.23, 1.08, 0.89, 0.86, 0.84 and 0.63 (each 3 H, s); between 2.90 and 3.80: glucose moiety with anomeric proton at 5,20 (1 H, d, *J* = 6.9 Hz, H-1′); ^{13}C-NMR (125 MHz; DMSO-d_6): δ 16.9, 24.5, 24.9 and 28.5; glucose moiety: 61.0, 69.9, 72.8, 77.1, 78.2, 94.5; 64.3 (C-23), 67.4 (C-2), 80.4 (C-3), 176.3 (C-28), 122.6 (C-12), 143.7 (C-13).

2α,3α,24-trihydroxyolean-11,13(18)-dien-28-oic acid. Yellowish powder; molecular formula $C_{30}H_{46}O_5$; ESI-MS: [M + Na]$^+$ *m/z* 509,375 (calc. 509,324) for $C_{30}H_{46}NaO_5$); ^{1}H-NMR(400 MHz; pyridin-d_5): δ 1.58; 1.06; 1.05; 1.03; 0.90 and 0.87 (each 3 H, s); 6.62 (1 H, d, *J* = 8.0 Hz, H-11) and 5.81 (1 H, d, *J* = 8.0 Hz, H-12); 4.38 (1 H, ddd, *J* =2.2; 7.6 and 8.9 Hz, H-2); 3.59 (1 H, d, *J* = 7.5 Hz, H-3); 4.43 (1 H, d, *J* = 8.7 Hz, H-24) and 3.75 (1 H, d, *J* = 8,76 Hz, H-24); 2.69 (1 H, d, *J* = 12.4 Hz, H-19) and 2.15 (1 H, d, *J* = 12.4 Hz, H-19); ^{13}C-NMR (125 MHz; pyridin-d_5): δ_C 16.6, 19.5, 19.8, 23.7, 24.0 and 32.1; 65.1 (C-24), 68.4 (C-2), 85.5 (C-3), 178,6 (C-28);136,1 (C-13); 133,3 (C-18); 126,4 (C-12) et 125,9 (C-11).

Apart from the activity profile described above, MIC values for the other tested fractions and compounds were above 39 μg/ml. The activity level of compounds 3,3′-di-O-methylellagic acid 4′-O-α-rhamnopyranoside and arjunglucoside was comparable to that of the reference drug fuconazole against *C. albicans*, and compound 3-O-methylellagic acid showed to be over 1.5 times more active than the same reference drug against *C. krusei*. Based on the basic skeleton of the tested compounds, it is important to notice that one of the most active derivatives, arjunglucoside and the less active compounds, arjungenin and 2α,3α,24-trihydroxyolean-11,13(18)-dien-28-oic acid are all triterpenoids. Preliminary structure-activity relationship (SAR) study clearly indicated that the glycosylation of the acidic function of arjungenin at C-28 is important for activity improvement. The other active compounds 3,3′-di-O-methylellagic acid 4′-O-α-rhamnopyranoside and 3-O-methylellagic acid are ellagic acid derivatives. Previous studies have reported the antifungal activity of ellagic acid against fungal strains *Trichophyton rubrum*, *T. verrucosum*, *T. mentagrophytes*, *T. violaceum*, *T. schoenleinii*, *Microsporum canis*, *C. glabrata*, *C. albicans* and *C. tropicalis* [41]. Also, the observed antifungal potency of compounds 3,3′-di-O-methylellagic acid 4′-O-α-rhamnopyranoside and 3-O-methylellagic acid, respectively glycosylated and methylated derivatives of ellagic acid, highlights the potency of this class of secondary metabolites [41].

Overall, it was observed that fraction T3 exerted the more potent effect against the tested yeasts, far better than the derived compounds. This is an indication that fractionation has declined the anti-yeast activity, emphasizing the relevance of potential synergistic interactions among the components of fraction T3. Moreover, these results indicate future directions in the progression of this fraction to develop a phytodrug against yeasts infections.

Selected isolated compounds were further tested against G6PD, carbonic anhydrase I, II and GST enzymes. The results achieved are shown in Table 2.

The G6PD enzyme was strongly inhibited by the triterpenoid arjunglucoside with IC_{50} value of 1.84 μM and Ki (the inhibitor constant indicating how potent an inhibitor is; or the concentration required to produce half maximum inhibition) value of 0.19 μM. It has been shown that this key metabolic enzyme which catalyzes the first step of the pentose phosphate pathway is expressed abundantly and is very active in human tumors [21]. In contrast, G6PD-deficient tumor cell lines showed relatively slow growth and enhanced apoptosis [42]. Previous studies also reported G6PD inhibitory properties for few compounds such as steroids and derivatives [43,44], chalcones [29], catechin gallates [45], and some phenolic molecules [46]. In this study, the substituted ellagic acid derived compound 3,3′-di-*O*-methylellagic acid 4′-*O*-α-rhamnopyranoside did not show any effect on the G6PD enzyme activity, although Adem et al. [46] had previously reported that ellagic acid inhibited the enzyme with an IC_{50} value of 0.072 mM. The methoxy group in this derivative may hinder the enzyme–inhibitor interaction. Based on the skeletal features of the tested triterpenoids—arjungenin, arjunglucoside, and 2α,3α,24-trihydroxyolean-11,13(18)-dien-28-oic acid—the presence of the hydroxyl group at C-19 and the glycosylation of the C-28 carboxylic group may be both factors of activity improvement. The G6PD inhibitory potential of a terpenoid is reported here for the first time.

Compound arjunglucoside exhibited very good potency against both CAI and CAII enzymes with respective activity parameters of IC_{50} = 3.28 μM and Ki = 2.72 μM; and IC_{50} = 1.28 μM and Ki = 1.03 μM respectively. The other tested compounds including 3,3′-di-*O*-methylellagic acid 4′-*O*-α-rhamnopyranoside and arjungenin were found to be moderately active against CAI and CAII (3,3′-di-*O*-methylellagic acid 4′-*O*-α-rhamnopyranoside) with IC_{50} and Ki values globally above 44 μM. Previous studies by Sarıkaya et al. [47] have indicated that ellagic acid inhibited CAI and CAII with K_i values of 0.207 and 0.146 mM respectively. In the present study, compound 3,3′-di-*O*-methylellagic acid 4′-*O*-α-rhamnopyranoside, a substituted derivative of ellagic acid has exhibited moderate, however highly improved potency toward CAI (K_i = 44.11 μM) and CAII (55.78 μM) enzymes. On the other hand, this substitution has also considerably decreased the activity as observed against the G6PD enzyme. In addition to the established role of CA inhibitors (CAIs) as diuretics and antiglaucoma drugs, it has recently emerged that they could have potential as novel anti-obesity, anticancer and anti-infective drugs [23]. The high inhibitory potency of the triterpenoid arjunglucoside against CAs indicates that it is a promising compound that might be a candidate for the formulation of drugs against CAIs-related diseases.

The screening of 3,3′-di-*O*-methylellagic acid 4′-*O*-α-rhamnopyranoside, arjungenin, and arjunglucoside against GST enzyme showed inhibitory effects. However, the triterpenoids arjungenin, and arjunglucoside exhibited highly potent inhibitory effects (IC_{50} of 1.57 and 1.84 μM respectively; and K_i of 1.00 and 1.23 μM respectively). Compound 3,3′-di-*O*-methylellagic acid 4′-*O*-α-rhamnopyranoside only exerted a moderate inhibitory effect on the enzyme (IC_{50} = 63.01 μM; K_i = 42.00 μM). These results are of higher significance as GST inhibitors are anti-cancer agents [25,26]. Ellagic acid was recently shown to inhibit GSTs A1-1, A2-2, M1-1, M2-2 and P1-1 with IC_{50} values ranging from 0.04 to 5 μM [48]. Preliminary SAR studies indicate that the substitution of ellagic acid at C-3 and C-4′ gave the derivative 3,3′-di-*O*-methylellagic acid 4′-*O*-α-rhamnopyranoside which showed an IC_{50} value of 63.01 μM, thus therefore considerably decreased the activity. The inhibitory effect of this class of secondary metabolite derivatives is reported here for the first time.

Table 2. Inhibitory parameters of isolated compounds against G6PD, CAI, CAII, and GST.

Activity	G6PD				CAI				CAII				GST			
Parameter	1	2	3	4	1	2	3	4	1	2	3	4	1	2	3	4
IC_{50} [a] (µM)	n.a	n.a	n.a	1.84 ± 0.31	53.31 ± 1.09		86.64 ± 0.93	3.28 ± 0.13	69.31 ± 1.13	n.a	n.a	1.03 ± 0.01	63.01 ± 1.15	n.a	1.51 ± 0.78	1.84 ± 0.73
Ki [b] (µM)	n.a	n.a	n.a	0.19 ± 0.03	44.11 ± 1.12		71.68 ± 0.96	2.72 ± 0.64	55.78 ± 0.97	n.a	n.a	1.84 ± 0.11	42.00 ± 1.39	n.a	1.00 ± 0.03	0.19 ± 0.77

Enzymes were expressed and purified, and subsequently assessed for in vitro susceptibility to inhibitors. [a] Serially diluted triplicate concentrations of compounds were tested and activity expressed as 50% inhibitory concentration; [b] Inhibitory constant which is reflective of the binding affinity; the smaller the Ki, the greater the binding affinity and the smaller amount of medication needed in order to inhibit the activity of that enzyme. n.a = non active. 1: 3,3′ di-O-methylellagic acid 4′-O-α-rhamnopyranoside; 2: 3-O-methylellagic acid; 3: arjungenin; 4: arjunglucoside. G6PD, glucose-6-phosphate dehydrogenase; CAI, human erythrocyte carbonic anhydrase I; CAII, human erythrocyte carbonic anhydrase II; GST, glutathione S-transferase.

5. Concluding Remarks

The results obtained from the investigation of the methanolic extract of *T. mantaly* stem bark have identified a highly potent anti-yeast fraction T3 that showed to be more promising than subsequently isolated compounds. Overall, the five compounds, 3,3′-di-*O*-methylellagic acid 4′-*O*-α-rhamnopyranoside, arjungenin, arjunglucoside, 2α,3α,24-trihydroxyolean-11,13(18)-dien-28-oic acid, and 3-*O*-methyl ellagic acid were found to be 243 to 31,250 times, 15 to 7,812 times, and 975 to 250,000 times less active than the mother fraction (T3) against *C. parapsilosis*, *C. albicans*, and *C. krusei* respectively. This promising fraction deserves to be further investigated with the ultimate aim of formulating a plant-based drug against yeast infections. Compounds 3,3′-di-*O*-methylellagic acid 4′-*O*-α-rhamnopyranoside and arjunglucoside showed anti-yeast activity close to that of the reference drug fuconazole against *C. albicans*. Moreover, compound 3-*O*-methyl ellagic acid was over 1.5 times more active than fuconazole against *C. krusei*. In addition, two of the islolated compounds, arjungenin and arjunglucoside were found to be very active against enzymes of metabolic significance, namely G6PD (arjunglucoside) and GST (arjungenin and arjunglucoside). Finally, given the anti-yeast potency of these compounds, and also the implication of the tested enzymes in some metabolic dysfunctions of public health significance (cancer, obesity, epilepsy), we envisage further SAR studies to identify potent hit derivatives that should subsequently enter the drug development pipeline.

Acknowledgments: The authors acknowledge the Alexander von Humboldt Foundation for providing a Fellowship to Bruno Ndjakou Lenta at Bielefeld University. Part of this study was supported by equipment from the Seeding Labs' Instrumental Access Grant (SL2012-2) to Fabrice Fekam Boyom.

Author Contributions: N.S., E.T., B.N.L., F.F.B. and S.A.N. designed and supervised the study; M.A.T.T., T.N.K., S.G., R.M.T.K., A.A., M.K., V.C. and R.D. performed the chemical and biological parts of the study and drafted the manuscript; B.N.L. and F.F.B. critically revised the manuscript. All authors agreed on the final version of the manuscript for submission to *Medicines*.

Conflicts of Interest: The authors declare no conflict of interest.

References

1. Arif, T.; Mandal, T.K.; Dabur, R. Natural products: Anti-fungal agents derived from Plants. In *Opportunity, Challenge and Scope of Natural Products in Medicinal Chemistry*; Pandalai, S.G., Ed.; Research Signpost: Trivandrum, India, 2011; pp. 283–311.

2. Nelesh, G. HIV-associated opportunistic fungal infections: A guide to using the clinical microbiology laboratory. *South. Arf. J. HIV Med.* **2007**, *1*, 18–23.

3. Álvaro-Meca, A.; Jensen, J.; Micheloud, D.; Asunción, D.; Gurbindo, D.; Resino, S. Rate of candidiasis among HIV infected children in Spain in the era of highly active antiretroviral therapy (1997–2008). *BMC Inf. Dis.* **2013**, *13*, 1–15. [CrossRef] [PubMed]

4. Brissaud, O.; Guichoux, J.; Harambat, J.; Tandonnet, O.; Zaoutis, T. Invasive fungal disease in PICU: Epidemiology and risk factors. *Ann. Intensiv. Care* **2012**, *2*. [CrossRef] [PubMed]

5. Ngouana, K.T.; Krasteva, D.; Drakulovski, P.; Toghueo, K.R.; Kouanfack, C.; Ambe, A.; Reynes, J.; Delaporte, E.; Boyom, F.F.; Mallié, M.; et al. Investigation of minor species *Candida africana*, *Candida stellatoidea*, and *Candida dubliniensis* in the *Candida albicans* complex among Yaoundé (Cameroon) HIV-infected patients. *Mycoses* **2015**, *58*, 33–39. [CrossRef] [PubMed]

6. Ngouana, K.T.; Dongtsa, J.; Kouanfack, C.; Tonfack, C.; Foména, S.; Krasteva, D.; Drakulovski, P.; Aghokeng, A.; Mallié, M.; Delaporte, E.; et al. Cryptoccocal meningitis in Yaoundé (Cameroon) HIV infected patients: Diagnosis, frequency and susceptibility of *Cryptococcus neoformans* isolates to fluconazole. *J. Mycol. Med.* **2015**, *25*, 11–16. [CrossRef] [PubMed]

7. Newman, D.J.; Cragg, G.M. Natural products as sources of new drugs over the last 25 years. *J. Nat. Prod.* **2007**, *70*, 461–477. [CrossRef] [PubMed]

8. Coulibaly, K. Evaluation of the Antifungal Activity of Extracts of Bark of Commercial Species, Category P1 the Forest of Mopri, Tiassalé (Southern Ivory Coast). Master's Thesis, University of Cocody-Abidjan, Abidjan, Côte D'Ivoire, 2006; pp. 23–25.

9. Ngouana, T.K.; Mbouna, C.D.J.; Kuipou, R.M.T.; Tchuenmogne, M.A.T.; Zeuko'o, E.M.; Ngouana, V.; Mallié, M.; Bertout, S.; Boyom, F.F. Potent and Synergistic Extract Combinations from *Terminalia Catappa*, *Terminalia Mantaly* and *Monodora tenuifolia* against Pathogenic Yeasts. *Medicines* **2015**, *2*, 220–235. [CrossRef]

10. Cock, I. The medicinal properties and phytochemistry of plants of the genus *Terminalia* (Combretaceae). *Inflammopharmacology* **2015**, *23*, 203–229. [CrossRef] [PubMed]

11. Valsaraj, R.; Pushpangadan, P.; Smitt, U.W.; Adersen, A.; Christensen, S.B.; Sittie, A.; Nyman, U.; Nielsen, C.; Olsen, C.E. New anti-HIV-1, antimalarial and antifungal compounds from *Terminalia bellerica*. *J. Nat. Prod.* **1997**, *60*, 739–742. [CrossRef] [PubMed]

12. Srivastava, S.K.; Srivastava, S.D.; Chouksey, B.K. New constituents of *Terminalia alata*. *Fitoterapia* **1999**, *70*, 390–394. [CrossRef]

13. Conrad, J.; Vogler, B.; Klaiber, I.; Roos, G.; Walter, U.; Kraus, W. Two triterpene esters from *Terminalia macroptera* bark. *Phytochemistry* **1998**, *48*, 647–650. [CrossRef]

14. Conrad, J.; Vogler, B.; Reeb, S.; Klaiber, I.; Papajewski, S.; Roos, G.; Vasquez, E.; Setzer, M.C.; Kraus, W. Isoterchebulin and 4,6-O-isoterchebuloyl-D-glucose, Novel Hydrolyzable Tannins from *Terminalia macroptera*. *J. Nat. Prod.* **2001**, *64*, 294–299. [CrossRef] [PubMed]

15. Kandil, F.E.; Nassar, M.I. A tannin anti-cancer promotor from *Terminalia arjuna*. *Phytochemistry* **1998**, *47*, 1567–1568. [CrossRef]

16. Mahato, S.B.; Nandy, A.K.; Kundu, A.H. Pentacyclic triterpenoids sapogenols and their glycosides from *Terminalia bellerica*. *Tetrahedron* **1992**, *48*, 2483–2484. [CrossRef]

17. Singh, D.V.; Verma, R.K.; Singh, C.S.; Gupta, M.M. RP-LC determination of oleane derivatives in *Terminalia arjuna*. *J. Pharm. Biomed. Anal.* **2002**, *28*, 447–452. [CrossRef]

18. Garcez, R.F.; Garcez, S.W.; Santana, A.L.B.D.; Alves, M.M.; Matos, M.F.C.C.; Scaliante, A.M. Bioactive flavonoids and triterpenes from *Terminalia fagifolia* (Combretaceae). *J. Braz. Chem. Soc.* **2006**, *17*, 1223–1228. [CrossRef]

19. Yeh, G.C.; Daschner, P.J.; Lopaczynska, J.; MacDonald, C.J.; Ciolino, H.P. Modulation of glucose-6-phosphate dehydrogenase activity and expression is associated with aryl hydrocarbon resistance in vitro. *J. Biol. Chem.* **2001**, *276*, 34708–34713. [CrossRef] [PubMed]

20. Matsubara, S.; Kato, T.; Oshikawa, K.; Yamada, T.; Takayama, T.; Koike, T.; Sato, I. Glucose-6-phosphate dehydrogenase in rat lung alveolar epithelial cells. An ultrastructural enzyme-cytochemical study. *Eur. J. Histochem.* **2002**, *46*, 243–248. [CrossRef] [PubMed]

21. Preuss, J.; Richardson, A.D.; Pinkerton, A.; Hedrick, M.; Sergienko, E.; Rahlfs, S.; Bode, L. Identification and characterization of novel human glucose-6-phosphate dehydrogenase inhibitors. *J. Biomol. Screen.* **2013**, *18*, 286–297. [CrossRef] [PubMed]

22. Tripp, B.C.; Smith, K.; Ferry, J.G. Mini review: Carbonic anhydrase: New insights for an ancient enzyme. *J. Biol. Chem.* **2001**, *276*, 48615–48618. [CrossRef] [PubMed]

23. Supuran, C.T. Carbonic anhydrases: Novel therapeutic applications for inhibitors and activators. *Nat. Rev. Drug Discov.* **2008**, *7*, 168–181. [CrossRef] [PubMed]

24. Comakli, V.; Ciftci, M.; Kufrevioglu, O.I. Effects of some metal ions on rainbow trout erythrocytes glutathione *S*-transferase enzyme: An in vitro study. *J. Enzyme Inhib. Med. Chem.* **2013**, *28*, 1261–1266. [CrossRef] [PubMed]

25. Mannervik, B.; Danielson, U.H. Glutathione transferases—Structure and catalitic activity. *CRC Crit. Rev. Biochem.* **1988**, *23*, 283–337. [CrossRef] [PubMed]

26. Matshushita, N.; Aritake, K.; Takada, A.; Hizue, M.; Hayashi, K.; Mitsui, K. Pharmacological studies on the novel antiallergenic drug HQL-79: 2. Elucidation of mechanisms for antiallergic and antiasthmatic effects. *Jpn. J. Pharmacol.* **1998**, *78*, 11–22. [CrossRef]

27. Hayes, J.D.; McLellan, L.I.; Stockman, P.K.; Chalmers, J.; Beckett, G.J. Glutathione *S*-transferases in man: The relationship between rat and human enzymes. *Biochem. Soc. Trans.* **1987**, *15*, 721–725. [CrossRef] [PubMed]

28. Mga'ning, B.M.; Lenta, B.N.; Noungoue, D.T.; Antheaume, C.; Fongang, Y.F.; Ngouela, S.A.; Boyom, F.F.; Rosenthal, P.J.; Tsamo, E.; Sewald, N.; et al. Antiplasmodial sesquiterpenes from the seeds of *Salacia longipes* var. *camerunensis*. *Phytochemistry* **2013**, *96*, 347–352. [CrossRef] [PubMed]

29. Kuzu, M.; Aslan, A.; Ahmed, I.; Comakli, V.; Demirdag, R.; Uzun, N. Purification of glucose-6-phosphate dehydrogenase and glutathione reductase enzymes from the gill tissue of Lake Van fish and analyzing the effects of some chalcone derivatives on enzyme activities. *Fish Physiol. Biochem.* **2016**, *42*, 483–491. [CrossRef] [PubMed]

30. Beutler, E. *Red Cell Metabolism: A Manual of Biochemical Methods*, 3rd ed.; Grune and Stratton Inc.: Orlando, FL, USA, 1984; pp. 68–70.

31. Ekinci, D.; Cavdar, H.; Talaz, O.; Sentürk, M.; Supuran, C.T. NO-releasing esters show carbonic anhydrase inhibitory action against human isoforms I and II. *Bioorg. Med. Chem.* **2010**, *18*, 3559–3563. [CrossRef] [PubMed]

32. Verpoorte, J.A.; Mehta, S.; Edsall, J.T. Esterase activities of human carbonic anhydrases B and C. *J. Biol. Chem.* **1976**, *242*, 4221–4229.

33. Hunaiti, A.A.; Soud, M. Effect of lead concentration on the level of glutathione, glutathione *S*-transferase, reductase and peroxidase in human blood. *Sci. Total Environ.* **2000**, *248*, 45–50. [CrossRef]

34. Güvercin, S.; Erat, M.; Sakiroglu, H. Determination of some kinetic and characteristic properties of glutathione *S*-transferase from bovine erythrocytes. *Protein Pept. Lett.* **2008**, *15*, 6–12. [PubMed]

35. Habig, W.H.; Pabst, M.J.; Jakoby, W.B. Glutathione *S*-transferases. The first enzymatic step in mercapturic acid formation. *J. Biol. Chem.* **1974**, *249*, 7130–7139. [PubMed]

36. Cheng, Y.; Prusoff, W.H. Relationship between the inhibition constant (K1) and the concentration of inhibitor which causes 50 per cent inhibition (I50) of an enzymatic reaction. *Biochem. Pharmacol.* **1973**, *22*, 3099–3108. [PubMed]

37. Liu, M.; Katerere, R.D.; Gray, I.A.; Seidel, V. Phytochemistry and antifungal studies on *Terminalia mollis* and *Terminalia brachystemina*. *Fitoterapia* **2009**, *80*, 369–373. [CrossRef] [PubMed]

38. Nandy, A.K.; Podder, G.; Sahu, N.P.; Mahato, S.B. Triterpenoids and their glycosides from *Terminalia bellerica*. *Phytochemistry* **1989**, *28*, 2769–2772. [CrossRef]

39. Jossang, A.; Seuleiman, M.; Maidou, E.; Bodo, B. Pentacyclic triterpenes from *Combretum nigricans*. *Phytochemistry* **1996**, *41*, 591–594. [CrossRef]

40. Kojima, H.; Tominaga, H.; Sato, S.; Ogura, H. Pentacyclic triterpenoids from *Prunella vulgaris*. *Phytochemistry* **1987**, *26*, 1107–1111. [CrossRef]

41. Li, Z.; Guo, X.; Dawuti, G.; Aibai, S. Antifungal activity of ellagic acid in vitro and in vivo. *Phytother. Res.* **2015**, *29*, 1019–1025. [CrossRef] [PubMed]

42. Kuo, W.Y.; Lin, J.Y.; Tang, K. Human glucose-6-phophate dehydrogenase (G6PD). Gene transforms NIH 3T3 cells and induces tumors in nude mice. *Int. J. Cancer* **2000**, *85*, 857–864. [CrossRef]

43. Gupta, S.; Cordeiro, T.A.; Michels, P.A.M. Glucose-6-phosphate dehydrogenase is the target for the trypanocidal action of human steroids. *Mol. Biochem. Parasitol.* **2011**, *176*, 112–115. [CrossRef] [PubMed]

44. Hamilton, M.N.; Dawson, M.; Fairweather, E.E.; Hamilton, S.N.; Hitchin, R.J.; James, I.D.; Jones, D.S.; Jordan, M.A.; Lyones, J.A.; Small, F.H. Novel steroid inhibitors of glucose 6-phosphate dehydrogenase. *J. Med. Chem.* **2012**, *55*, 4431–4445. [CrossRef] [PubMed]

45. Shin, E.S.; Park, J.; Shin, J.M.; Cho, D.; Cho, S.Y.; Shin, D.W.; Ham, M.; Kim, J.B.; Lee, T.R. Cathechin gallates are NADP⁺-competitive inhibitors of glucose-6-phosphate dehydrogenase and other enzymes that employ NADP⁺ as a coenzyme. *Bioorg. Med. Chem.* **2008**, *16*, 3580–3586. [CrossRef] [PubMed]

46. Adem, S.; Comakli, V.; Kuzu, M.; Demirdag, R. Investigation of the effects of some phenolic compounds on the Activities of glucose-6-phosphate dehydrogenase and 6-Phosphogluconate dehydrogenase from human erythrocytes. *J. Biochem. Mol. Toxicol.* **2014**, *28*, 510–514. [CrossRef] [PubMed]

47. Beyza, Ö.S.; Gülçin, İ.; Supuran, C.T. Carbonic anhydrase inhibitors: Inhibition of human erythrocyte isozymes I and II with a series of phenolic acids. *Chem. Biol. Drug Des.* **2010**, *75*, 515–520. [CrossRef] [PubMed]

48. Hayeshi, R.; Mutingwende, I.; Mavengere, W.; Masiyanise, V.; Mukanganyama, S. The inhibition of human glutathione *S*-transferases activity by plant polyphenolic compounds ellagic acid and curcumin. *Food Chem. Toxicol.* **2007**, *45*, 286–295. [CrossRef] [PubMed]

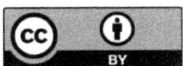

medicines   【MDPI】

Article

Isolation and Cytotoxic Investigation of Flacourtin from *Oncoba spinosa*

Olaoye S. Balogun *, Olukayode S. Ajayi and Olayinka S. Lawal

Department of Chemistry, Obafemi Awolowo University, Ile-Ife 220005, Nigeria; osajayi@oauife.edu.ng (O.S.A.); lawalolayinka@gmail.com (O.S.L.)
* Correspondence: solomonoye@gmail.com or balogunolaoye@oauife.edu.ng; Tel.: +234-803-494-0850

Academic Editor: James D. Adams
Received: 26 October 2016; Accepted: 29 November 2016; Published: 6 December 2016

Abstract: Background: *Oncoba spinosa*, an endangered medicinal plant whose secondary metabolites have not been extensively profiled, and which is hitherto yet to be examined for cytotoxicity, is being investigated in this study. **Methods:** Leaves of *Oncoba spinosa* (800 g) were extracted with 95% aqueous methanol. The crude extract was partitioned with n-hexane and the resultant defatted extract was extensively chromatographed on silica gel to yield compound **1** which was subjected to spectroscopic analysis. A brine shrimps lethality test was used to establish the cytotoxicity potentials of the isolated compound and the plant extracts. **Results:** Compound **1** was elucidated as flacourtin, 3-hydroxy-4-hydroxymethylphenyl-6-O-benzoyl-β-D-glucopyranoside. The LD_{50} values obtained were less than 1000 μg/mL for flacourtin and the plant extracts. **Conclusion:** Flacourtin is being reported for the first time in the *O. spinosa*. The preliminary toxicity assay indicated that flacourtin and the plant extracts were not cytotoxic; thus, the tradomedicinal uses of the plant may portend no danger.

Keywords: *Oncoba spinosa*; Flacourtin; cytotoxicity; Flacourtiaceae; phenolic ester glycoside

1. Introduction

O. spinosa is a spiny shrub used for the management of arthritis in southwest Nigeria [1]. The fruit is used for the treatment of anthelminthic, syphilis, wound and sexual impotence [2]. In profiling the chemical constituent of *Oncoba spinosa*, (Flacourtiaceae) five flavonoids, kaempferol, quercetin, apigenin-7-O-β-D-glucuronopyranoside, quercetin 3-O-β-D-galactopyranoside and quercetin 3-O-α-rhamnopyranosyl (1→6) β-D-glucopyranoside have been reported [3]. Flacourtin, a phenolic glycoside ester (3-hydroxy-4-hydroxymethylphenyl-6-O-benzoyl-β-D-glucopyranoside) which has been associated with a number of pharmacological activities was first isolated from the bark of a medicinal plant, *Flacourtia indica* (Flacourtiaceae) [4–8], an indigenous medicinal plant widely distributed in India and Bangladesh [9]. Also, Amarasinghe et al. [10] reported isolation of a new glucoside, flacourside, an analog of flacourtin from *Flacourtia indica*. As part of our on-going work on metabolite profiling of indigenous medicinal plants, leaves of *O. spinosa* were collected with the aim of isolating a bioactive compound new to the plant specie.

2. Materials and Methods

2.1. Plant Collection and Purification

Fresh leaves *Oncoba spinosa* were collected at the Botanical Garden University of Ibadan, Oyo State, Nigeria in the month of November, 2014. The plant was identified by the taxonomist and curator, Mr A. Owolabi in the Botanical Garden. A voucher copy of the plant with herbarium number FHI 108806 was deposited at the Forestry Research Institute of Nigeria, Ibadan.

The air-dried and pulverized leaves (800 g) were extracted with 95% aqueous methanol to give a crude extract (140 g). The crude was reconstituted in methanol and defatted with n-hexane to afford 80.60 g of defatted extract. Twenty grams of the defatted extract was chromatographed on silica gel using gradient of dichloromethane and methanol to give a sub-fraction (1.22 g) which was further purified on silica with gradient of hexane, ethyl acetate and methanol. Compound **1** (6 mg) was obtained as an off-white powder which was recrystallized in ethylacetate and thereafter subjected to spectroscopic analysis.

2.2. Cytotoxicity Assay

Cytotoxicity of the crude extract, defatted fraction and compound **1** were investigated using brine shrimp lethality assay. A spoonful quantity of the egg of brine shrimps (*Artemia salina* Leach) was sprinkled into a partly covered crucible containing seawater in order to allow partial illumination. The eggs hatched into matured *nauplii* after about 48 h and 10 matured *nauplii* were added to varying concentration of the test samples (1000, 100 and 10 μg/mL). All the experiments were carried out in triplicate and distilled water was used in place of the test samples for negative control. Numbers of survivors were counted after 24 h and the LC_{50} was computed at 95% confidence limit using the Finney program.

3. Results

IR ν_{max} (cm^{-1}): 3000 (ArO–H str), 3050 (Ar–H str), 1710 (C=O str), 1600 (Ar C–C str), 1220 (C–O ester), 1053 (C–O alc).

^{13}C-NMR (MeOD, 75 MHz): δc 134.5 ($C_{-1'}$), 130.7 ($C_{-2'}$ and $C_{-6'}$), 129.7 ($C_{-3'}$ and $C_{-5'}$), 132 ($C_{-5'}$), 150.1 ($C_{-1''}$), 116.3 ($C_{-2''}$), 154 ($C_{-3''}$), 134.1 ($C_{-4''}$), 115.7 ($C_{-5''}$), 119.7 ($C_{-6''}$), 61.1 ($C_{-7''}$), 104.6 (C_{-1}), 75.7 (C_{-2}), 75.2 (C_{-3}), 72.1(C_{-4}), 78.1 (C_{-5}), 64.8 (C_{-6}), 182 (C=O).

^{1}H-NMR (MeOD, 300 MHz): δ 8.05 (2H, m, J_o 7.2 Hz, J_m 1.5 Hz, H_{-2} and H_{-6}), 7.53 (2H, m, $J_{3,2}$ 7.2 Hz, $J_{3,5}$ 7.8 Hz , H_{-3} and H_{-5}), 7.66 (1H, m, J_o 7.5 Hz, J_m 1.5 Hz, H_{-5}), 6.77 (1H, d, J_m 3.0 Hz, $H_{-2''}$), 7.03 (1H, d, J_o 8.7 Hz, $H_{-5''}$), 6.48 (1H, dd, J_o 8.7 Hz, J_m 3.3 Hz, $H_{-6''}$), 4.62 (1H, d, H_{-1}), 3.51 (3H, m, H_{-2}, H_{-3} and H_{-4}), 3.73 (1H, m, $J_{5,6}$ 7.5 Hz, H_{-5}), 4.46 (1H, d, $J_{5,6}$ 7.5 Hz, H_{-6a}), 4.42 (IH, d, $J_{5,6}$ 7.5 Hz, H_{-6b}), 4.72 (H, $H_{-6a''}$), 4.76 (1H, $H_{-6b''}$), 4.95, 4.82 and 4.72 (glucose OH), 4.69 (benzylic OH).

4. Discussion

The NMR spectra of compound **1** showed a pattern characteristic of a phenolic ester glycoside. Clusters of peaks at δ 3.5–5.0 indicated the presence of a sugar moiety while the aromatic region showed the presence of eight protons with *J* values typical of an aromatic system, thus suggesting two substituted benzene rings (Figure 1). The IR spectrum showed absorption bands (cm^{-1}) at 3000 (ArO–H str), 3050 (Ar–H str), 1710 (C=O str), 1600 (Ar C–C str), 1220 (C–O ester), 1053 (C–O alc) and 810 (1,2,4-trisubstituted aromatic). The chemical shift δ 61.1–78.1 ppm in the ^{13}C-NMR spectrum indicated *O*-linked carbons of the sugar moiety and the carbinol carbon of the phenolic aglycone. The anomeric carbon and the carbonyl of ester resonated at δ 104.6 and 182 ppm respectively while the aromatic carbons were observed at δ 115.7–150.1 ppm. The spectrum of ^{1}H NMR indicated a multiplet at δ 3.50 assignable to three methine protons on the glucose moiety and two doublets of carbinol protons at δ 4.46 (1H, d, $J_{5,6}$ 7.5 Hz) and δ 4.42 (IH, d, $J_{5,6}$ 7.5 Hz) coupling with H_{-5} at δ 3.73 ppm (1H, m, $J_{5,6}$ 7.5 Hz). The anomeric proton appeared as a doublet at δ 4.62 ppm indicating an axial position to the pyranose ring.

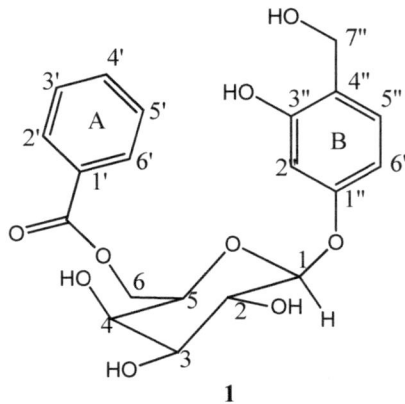

Figure 1. Flacourtin.

Three aromatic protons of ring B with *J* values attributable to a 1,2,4-trisubstituted aromatic system showed at δ 7.03, 6.77 and 6.48. The two protons each at ortho and meta position in ring A are in the same chemical environment, thus both protons at ortho position resonated at δ 8.05 with J_o and J_m of 7.2 and 1.5 Hz respectively. Similarly, symmetrical protons at meta positions were observed at δ 7.53 with coupling constant of 7.2 and 7.8 Hz, showing that the protons were doubly ortho-coupled, which connoted that ring A is monosubstituted. All the spectroscopic data and their assignments were in good agreement with the report of Bhaumik et al. [4]. The compound (Figure 1), which was isolated for the first time from leaves of *O. spinosa*, was elucidated as 3-hydroxy-4-hydroxymethylphenyl-6-*O*-benzoyl-β-D-glucopyranoside, previously named flacourtin.

The brine shrimps lethality test indicated that crude extract, methanol fraction and flacourtin had LD_{50} values greater than 1000 μg/mL (Table 1) which implied that they exhibited no cytotoxic activity on the *nauplii*.

Table 1. Cytotoxicity of test samples.

Sample	Crude	n-Hexane Fraction	Defatted Fraction	Flacourtin
LD_{50} (μg/mL)	1203	>10,000	>10,000	>10,000

5. Conclusions

Flacourtin is being reported for the first time in the *O. spinosa*. The preliminary toxicity profile as indicated by brine shrimp lethality test showed that the compound and the plant extracts were not cytotoxic; therefore, the tradomedicinal uses of the plant may portend no danger.

Author Contributions: Olaoye S. Balogun conceived and designed the experiment with Olukayode S. Ajayi while Lawal S. Olayinka performed the experiment.

Conflicts of Interest: The authors declare no conflict of interest.

References

1. Gbadamosi, I.T.; Oloyede, A.A. Mineral, proximate and phytochemical components of ten Nigeria medicinal plants used in the management of arthritis. *Afr. J. Pharm. Pharmacol.* **2014**, *8*, 638–643. [CrossRef]
2. Ramzi, A.; Mothana, A.; Kriegisch, S.; Harms, M.; Kristian, W.; Landequist, U. Assessment of Yemeni medinal plant for their in vitro antimicrobial, anticancer, and antioxidant activities. *J. Pharm. Biol.* **2011**, *49*, 200–210.

3. Djoussi, M.G.; Jean, D.M.; David, N.; Jules, R.K.; Leon, A.T.; Dominique, H.; Laurence, V.N. Antimicrobial and antioxidant flavonoids from the leaves of *Oncoba spinosa*. *BMC Complement. Altern. Med.* **2005**, *15*, 134. [CrossRef] [PubMed]
4. Bhaumik, P.K.; Guha, K.P.; Biswas, G.K.; Mukherjee, B. (−)Flacourtin, a phenolic glucoside ester from *Flacourtia indica*. *Phytochemistry* **2005**, *26*, 3090–3091. [CrossRef]
5. Nazneen, M.; Mazid, M.A.; Kundu, J.K.; Bachar, S.C.; Begum, F.; Datta, B.K. Protective effects of *Flacourtia indica* aerial parts extracts against paracetamol-induced hepatotoxiciy in rats. *J. Taibah Univ. Sci.* **2009**, *2*, 1–6. [CrossRef]
6. Saxena, A.; Patel, B.D. In vitro antioxidant activity of methanolic and aqueous extract of *Flacourtia indica* Merr. *Am.-Eurasian J. Sci. Res.* **2010**, *5*, 201–206.
7. Singh, T.S.; Singh, M.; Yadav, D.; Singh, I.; Mansoori, M.H. Antiasthmatic potential of *Flacourtia indica* Merr. *Afr. J. Basic Appl. Sci.* **2011**, *3*, 201–204.
8. Eramma, N.; Gayathri, D. Antibacterial potential and phytochemical analysis of *Flacourtia indica* (Burm.f.) Merr. root extract against human pathogens. *Indo Am. J. Pharm. Res.* **2013**, *3*, 3832–3846.
9. Patro, S.K.; Behera, P.C.; Kumar, P.M.; Sasmal, D.; Padhy, R.K.; Dash, S.K. Pharmacological Review of *Flacourtia sepiaria* (Ruxb.). *Sch. Acad. J. Pharm.* **2013**, *2*, 89–93.
10. Amarasinghe, N.R.; Jayasinghe, L.; Hara, N.; Fujimoto, Y. Flacourside, a new 4-oxo-2-cyclopentenylmethyl glucoside from the fruit juice of *Flacourtia indica*. *Food Chem.* **2007**, *102*, 95–97. [CrossRef]

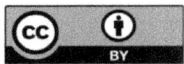

medicines

MDPI

Article

Chemical Composition, Cytotoxic, Apoptotic and Antioxidant Activities of Main Commercial Essential Oils in Palestine: A Comparative Study

Mohammad A. Al-Tamimi [1,*], Bob Rastall [2] and Ibrahim M. Abu-Reidah [1,3]

1   Deptartment of Nutrition and Food Technology, An-Najah National University, PO Box 7, Nablus 415, Palestine
2   Department of Food and Nutritional Sciences, The University of Reading, Whiteknights, Reading RG6 6AP, UK; r.a.rastall@reading.ac.uk
3   Deptartment of Chemistry, An-Najah National University, PO Box 7, Nablus 415, Palestine; iabureidah@gmail.com or iabureidah@najah.edu
*   Correspondence: m.altamimi@najah.edu; Tel.: +970-595591255

Academic Editor: James D. Adams
Received: 1 September 2016; Accepted: 19 October 2016; Published: 25 October 2016

Abstract: Background: Essential oils (EOs) are complex mixtures of several components gifted with a wide array of biological activities. The present research was designed to evaluate whether commercial essential oils could be effective by examining their in vitro antioxidant, cytotoxic, and apoptotic properties of nine commercially available EOs in Palestine, namely, African rue, basil, chamomile, fennel, fenugreek, ginger, spearmint, sage, and thyme, and to assure their effective use. **Methods:** The cytotoxic activity was determined using HT29-19(A) non-muco secreting and HT29-muco secreting (MS) cell lines. MTT, and trypan blue tests, and DPPH radical scavenging have also been assayed on the studied EOs. **Results:** In this work chamomile oil showed the lowest IC_{50} at the content of 60 µL/mL, while all other EOs reached such a decrease when 70–80 µL/mL was used on HT-29 (MS) cell lines. In HT-29 19(A) cells, 50% of viability was obtained when 80 µL/mL of ginger and African rue was used, while all other EOs needed more than 80 µL/mL to reach such a decline in viability. Otherwise, an MTT assay on HT-29 (MS) displayed ginger EO with the lowest IC_{50}, followed by African rue and sage, with 40, 48 and 53 µL/mL, respectively. Otherwise, for the rest of the EOs, the IC_{50} was obtained by assaying around 80 µL/mL. Ginger showed the lowest IC_{50} with 60 µL/mL and thyme was the highest with 77 µL/mL when HT-29 19(A) cells were used. **Conclusion:** The most active EOs were found to be ginger, chamomile oil, and African rue. In general, the results demonstrate that most commercial EOs tested in this work possess low, or no biological activities; this may be due to processing, storage conditions, and handling or other reasons, which may cause losses in the biological and pharmacological properties that endemically exist in the Eos; hence, more investigation is still required on commercial EOs before they are recommended to the public.

Keywords: essential oils (EOs); cytotoxicity; apoptosis; antioxidants; cell lines; anti-cancer activity

1. Introduction

Aromatic plants (APs) have been used since antiquity as a potential source of drug discovery and development of disease chemoprevention, in folk medicine, and as preservatives in foods [1]. The best known aromatic plants: viz, chamomile, fennel, ginger, thyme, basil, and sage, originate from the Mediterranean area. The Middle East in general and Palestine in particular, are areas with many endemic plants whose compounds could be used in medicine [2,3]. Many APs are used for different industrial purposes such as food, drugs, and perfumery manufacturing.

APs contain many biologically active compounds, mainly phenolics and EOs, which have been found to possess antioxidant, antiparasitic, antimicrobial, anti-carcinogenic, and anti-inflammatory properties, among others [4]. Essential oils (EOs) are also used for the management of chronic diseases like cardiovascular, diabetes, Alzheimer's, cancer, and others [5].

EOs are natural, concentrated, volatile aromatic compounds isolated from plants which have long been used in medicine, pharmaceutical, perfumery, cosmetic, and in many food applications. Initially, EOs have been utilized in medicine, but in the last decades their use as fragrance and essence ingredients has improved to become the major employment. Up to now, about 3000 EOs are well-known, of which, around 10% is engaged commercially in the flavor and aroma markets [6].

It is well-known that EOs are found in lots of APs, which possess a wide array of biological and pharmacological activities, which are associated with traditional and complementary medicine [4].

EOs are highly complex mixtures involving several tens to hundreds of different types of individual volatile compounds such as terpenoid, oxygenated terpenes, sesquiterpenes, and hydrocarbons, which are responsible for their characteristic aroma. EOs are hydrophobic liquids with a particular odor and taste aroma which are often poorly soluble in water. EOs have been widely used for their virucidal, bactericidal, fungicidal, anticancer, antioxidant, antidiabetic activities [7,8]. They are usually prepared by fragrance extraction techniques such as distillation (hydro or steam distillation), cold pressing, extraction (maceration), or by using of supercritical carbon dioxide extraction [9,10]. The biological activity of EOs is strictly linked to their chemical composition.

Table 1 presents a list of common EOs commercially available in Palestine and their sources.

Commercial EOs are of great interest for consumers with people being prescribed them as traditional remedies. Doses of 5 to 20 mL of EOs can be prescribed to people to relieve pains, headaches, joint arthritis and problems in the digestive system (personal observation).

Indeed, there is a relationship between the production of reactive oxygen species (ROS) to the origin of oxidation and inflammation that can lead to cancer [11]. Oxidative stress is a major contributor to the pathogenesis of a number of chronic diseases, that is why antioxidant behavior is one of the most commonly determined biological activities in extracts of plants such as EOs [12]. It has been reported that more than half of most cancer cases and their consequent deaths worldwide are potentially preventable [13]. Therefore, modification in dietary habits by increasing consumption of functional foods rich in antioxidants such as EOs is greatly supported [14].

The anticancer activity of EOs has been described in more than five hundred scientific reports; those first published dated to the 1960s [15].

So far, the effects of EOs have been investigated on glioblastoma, melanoma, leukemia and oral cancers, as well as on bone, breast, cervix, colon, lung, prostate, and uterus cancers [16]. Among the anticancer medications, 70% of drugs approved between 1940 and 2002 are either natural products or developed based on knowledge gained from natural products [17]. Most researchers who experimented on the anti-proliferation properties of natural compounds have examined the apoptosis process of certain cancer cells [18].

In spite of all the information available on several EOs, the investigation dealing with this kind of commercial product has been inadequate. Moreover, to the best of our knowledge, there are no reports available about in vitro cytotoxicity of these studied commercial EOs against HT29-19A non-muco secreting and HT29-muco secreting cell line types. Therefore, the aim of the present work has been to study and compare the antioxidant, cytotoxic, and apoptotic activities of nine commercially available EOs together with their in vitro anticancer activity assayed by methyl thiazol tetrazolium (MTT) and trypan blue tests, in order to evaluate their significance for traditional use.

Table 1. A list of the main popular commercial EOs in Palestine.

Essential Oil	Plant Family	Traditional Use and Activity	Reference
African rue (*Peganum harmala* L.)	Nitrariaceae (Zygophyllaceae)	Coughs, hypertension, diabetes, asthma, jaundice, lumbago, and many other human ailments, skin and subcutaneous tumors, skin diseases, wounds and lice.	[10,19]
Basil (*Ocimum basilicum* L.)	Lamiaceae	Antifungal, physicochemical and insect-repelling activity, antiseptic (postpartum infections) depression, migraine, stomach and intestinal ache.	[11]
Chamomile (*Matricaria chamomilla* L.)	Asteraceae	Abscesses, allergies, arthritis, boils, colic, cuts, cystitis, dermatitis, dysmenorrhea, earache, flatulence, hair, headache, inflamed skin, insect bites, insomnia, nausea, neuralgia, PMS, rheumatism, sores, sprains, strains, stress, wounds.	[12]
Fennel (*Foeniculum vulgare* Mill.)	Apiaceae (Umbelliferae)	Fennel essential oil is used as flavoring agents in food products also used as a constituent in cosmetic and pharmaceutical products. Herbal drugs and essential oil of fennel have antispasmodic, diuretic, anti-inflammatory, analgesic and antioxidant effects are active for dyspeptic complaints, flatulence and bloating. The volatile oil showed antimicrobial and hepatoprotective activity.	[13]
Fenugreek (*Trigonellafoenum-graecum* L.)	Fabaceae	Diabetes, sexual weakness, stomach and intestinal pain. The oil in the seeds is used as a skin softener and emollient. Fenugreek essential oil is rich in terpenenes.	[14,15]
Ginger (*Zingiber officinale* R.)	Zingiberaceae	wide application in flavor and perfumery industries, anti-emetic effect or control of nausea and vomiting, prevention of coronary artery disease, healing and prevention of both arthritic conditions and stomach ulcers.	[16]
Spearmint (*Mentha spicata* L.)	Lamiaceae	Food, cosmetic, confectionary, chewing gum, toothpaste and pharmaceutical industries. strong insecticidal and mutagenic activity.	[17]
Sage (*Salvia fruticosa* Mill.)	Lamiaceae	Antibacterial, cytostatic, antiviral and antioxidant activities. Moreover, they are frequently used in traditional medicine to treat diarrhea, eye diseases, gonorrhea; they possess antiseptic and antispasmodic activities. Also, the essential oils of Salvia species are used as cosmetics and as flavoring agents in perfumery.	[18]
Thyme (*Thymus vulgaris* L.)	Lamiaceae	Natural antimutagen	[20]

2. Materials and Methods

2.1. Essential Oils

The following commercial EOs were purchased from a local market in the city of Tulkarm, Palestine in May 2015, which was the end of the season for most aromatic plants grown locally, without knowing the conditions of production of these EOs. They are: African rue, basil, chamomile, fennel, fenugreek, ginger, mint, sage, and thyme, which are widely used in Palestine. All oils were micro-filtered using 0.2 μM disc (Sartorius Stedim Biotech, Goettingen, Germany) in order to eliminate any impurity present in the EO, then EOs were kept at 4 °C in dark containers till they were used for the experiment.

2.2. Gas Chromatography-Mass Spectrometry (GC-MS)

The analysis of the commercial EOs was performed on a GC-MS HP model 5975B inert MSD (Agilent Technologies, J&W Scientific Products, Palo Alto, CA, USA), equipped with an Agilent Technologies capillary DB-5MS column (30 m length; 0.25 mm i.d.; 0.25 mm film thickness), and coupled to a mass selective detector (MSD5975B, ionization voltage 70 eV; all Agilent, Santa Clara, CA, USA). The carrier gas (He) was used at a 1 mL min^{-1} flow rate. The oven temperature program was as follows: 1 min at 100 °C ramped from 100 to 260 °C at 4 °C min^{-1} and 10 min at 260 °C. The component concentration was obtained by semi-quantification by peak area integration from GC peaks.

2.3. Cell Culture Maintenance and Preparation

Mucus-secreting HT29-MS and non-mucus-secreting HT29-A (19) cells were obtained from the cells and culture collection at the University of Reading, UK. All cells were cultured in Dulbecco's modified Eagle medium (DMEM)-high glucose, contains sodium pyruvate (Life Technologies, Paisley, UK), supplemented with 10% defibrinated fetal bovine serum, 5% GlutaMAX™ (Life Technologies, Paisley, UK) and 1% antibacterial/antimycotic solution (Sigma-Aldrich, Pool, UK). All cells were grown in T-75 cm^2 flask and incubated at 37 °C with 5% CO_2 and 95% relative humidity. Media were changed every other day.

After reaching 70%–80% confluence, cells were split as follows; media were aspirated and cells were washed twice with 5 mL pre-warmed Phosphate buffered saline (Sigma-Aldrich, Pool, UK), then 5 mL trypsin-EDTA (0.5 g/L, Sigma-Aldrich, Pool, UK) was added and cells were re-incubated for a further 10 min. Trypsin was deactivated by adding 5 mL fresh medium and the suspension was centrifuged at 1800 rpm for 5 min. Supernatant was aspirated, then pelleted cells were reconstituted with 1 mL fresh medium. Cell count was conducted using a hemocytometer and microscopy and 105 cells/mL were recultured in a sterile flask. Flasks were monitored daily and checked microscopically for any contamination.

For the experiment, cells were cultured as above for 21 days and 15 days for HT29-(MS) and HT29-19 (A), respectively, so they reach maturation then they were used for viability, cytotoxicity and apoptosis tests.

2.4. Trypan Blue Exclusion Assay

To determine the effect of the EOs on the viability of cells, approximately, 105 mature cells/mL were transferred in a 12-well tissue culture plate and left for 48 h to establish adherence to plate before different concentrations of EOs were mixed with DMEM media and 500 μL/mL of such mixture were pipetted into each well. Some wells with media containing no EOs were used as control. After 24 h the media were aspirated and cells were trypsinized, collected and resuspended in an equivolume of 0.4% Trypan blue (Sigma-Aldrich, Pool, UK). This experiment was done in triplicates and repeated three times. The percentages of viable cells were counted using an inverted microscope and the percent of viability was determined in comparison with the control. Photos for cells under the microscope at different time intervals were taken using a Nikon™ Coolpix, 5400 digital camera (Nikon Inc., Melville, NY, USA).

2.5. MTT Cytotoxicity Assay

The in vitro cytotoxic activity of the EOs on HT29-19 (A) and HT29-(MS) was determined using the MTT (3-[4,5-dimethylthiazol-2-yl]-2,5-diphenyl tetrazolium bromide) assay as follows. Briefly, 200 μL/mL of medium containing cells at a density of 2×105 mature cells/mL were seeded in each well of a flat-bottom 96-well plate. Cells were permitted to adhere to the plate for 48 h. Then media were replaced with 180 μL/mL of various concentrations of the EOs (0%–100% of original EOs mixed with DMEM media) and incubated for 24 h. After that, MTT solution (0.5 mg/mL, Sigma-Aldrich) 20 μL/mL was added. Plates were incubated at 37 °C for another 4 h after which cultures were removed from incubator and the resulting formazan crystals were dissolve by adding an amount of MTT solubilizing solution (10% Triton X-100 with 0.1 N HCl in anhydrous isopropanol) equal to the original culture medium volume. All tests and analyses were run in triplicate. Pipetting up and down was required to completely dissolve the MTT formazan crystals. DMSO was used as the positive control and wells were left with no cells for the negative control. The absorbance of each well was determined by a spectrophotometer at dual wavelengths of 570 and 690 nm for the background on a multi-well plate reader with software (Tecan Group Ltd., Mannedorf, Switzerland). The viability percentage was calculated by the following formula: the concentration providing 50% inhibition (IC_{50}) was calculated from a graph plotting inhibition percentage against different EOs concentration.

Each experimental condition was analyzed in triplicate, with three experiments for each EO. Growth inhibition was calculated as follows:

$$\% \text{ Viability} = (OD_{sample} - OD_{blank}/OD_{control} - OD_{blank}) \times 100$$

2.6. DPPH Radical Scavenging Assay

DPPH (2,2-Diphenyl-1-picrylhydrazyl, Sigma-Aldrich, Pool, UK) radical scavenging activity was measured as described by Molyneux [21] with some modifications. Briefly, 0.5 mL of EO (8 mg/mL in methanol) was added to 1 mL of DPPH solution (20 mg/mL in methanol) freshly prepared. After shaking, the mixture was incubated for 15 min in darkness at room temperature and then absorbance was measured at 517 nm against a control (mixture without EO). Quercetin (Sigma-Aldrich, Pool, UK) was used as positive control. The inhibition percentage of free DPPH radicals (I%) was calculated following the formula:

$$\text{Percentage of radical scavenging} = (Abs_{control} - (Abs_{sample}/Abs_{control})) \times 100$$

where $Abs_{control}$ is the absorbance of the control reaction (blank with methanol and DPPH) and Abs_{sample} is the absorbance of the sample reaction (essential oil diluted in methanol and DPPH). The sample concentration (in 1 mL reaction mixture) providing 50% inhibition was estimated by plotting the percentages of inhibition against essential oil concentrations (Table 2). All determinations were performed in triplicate.

Table 2. DPPH Scavenging activity of the tested EOs.

Commercial EOs	African Rue	Basil	Chamomile	Fennel	Fenugreek	Ginger	Mint	Sage	Thyme
Quercetin equivalent (μg/mL)	20	20	20	20	<20	<20	<20	<20	<20

Five hundred µL of EO (8 mg/mL in methanol) was added to 1 mL of DPPH solution (20 mg/mL in methanol) freshly prepared. After shaking, the mixture was incubated for 15 min in darkness at room temperature and then absorbance was measured at 517 nm against a control. Quercetin was used for comparison.

2.7. Apoptosis Assay

Depending on cytotoxicity results, ginger oil was selected for examining apoptosis property which was measured using caspase-3 activity kit (Abcam, Cambridge, UK) according to the instructions of the manufacturer. Briefly, apoptosis was induced in cells by adding ginger oil, and the cells were incubated for 2 h. In addition, a control culture without induction was concurrently incubated. Cells were pelleted and counted almost 1×10^6 cells. Cells were also re-suspended in 50 µL of chilled cell lysis buffer and incubated on ice for 10 min. Finally, they were centrifuged for 1 min in a micro-centrifuge ($10,000 \times g$).

3. Results

3.1. EOs Composition

For the used commercial oils, the supplier provided no data about their contents or chemical analysis, which is presumed to be the company's copyright. However, a simple chemical analysis was performed in order to have a gross estimate of the components of the employed essential oils as % composition (Table 3).

Table 3. Main chemical components of the investigated EOs using GC-MS.

Components of EOs	A. Rue (%)	Basil (%)	Chamomile (%)	Fennel (%)	Fenugreek (%)	Ginger (%)	Mint (%)	Sage (%)	Thyme (%)
(E)-Anethol	13								
Eugenol	20								
Cicloysosativene	5								
3-Decanone	1								
α-Isomethyl-(E)-ionol	7								
Carvone	2						80		
Carvacrol	6								8
Dihydrocarvenyl acetate							1		
Caryophyllene	3	1			15		1		
Neral (cis-citral)					17	9			
Methyl chavicol		76							
Limonene	1						9		15
Linalool		15							
Thymol	7								25
ρ-Cymene									14
α-Pinene				1	2		0.5		12
β-Pinene					15				
Anethole				75					
Fenchone				13					
Cis-thujone								30	
Camphor	3				17			22	
1,8-Cineole								8	
α-Selinene					4.5				
Geranial					5	10			
2,5-Dimethylpyrazine					7				
α-Bisabolol oxide A			24						
Chamazulene			10						
α-Bisabolone oxide A			19						
α-Bisabolol oxide B			30						
Spathulenol			4						
α-Zingiberene						17.4			
Camphene						8			
α-Farnesene						6			
β-Sesquiphellandrene						6.6			
Total identified chemicals	66%	92%	87%	89%	82.5%	57%	91.5%	60%	74%

3.2. Viability Test by Trypan Blue

Viability test of both cell lines by trypan blue is shown in Figure 1a,b. HT-29 (MS) cell line viability decreased by 50% when 60 µL/mL of chamomile were used while all other EOs reached such a decrease when 70–80 µL/mL were used. In HT-29 19(A), 50% of viability was obtained when using 80 µL/mL of ginger and African rue, while all other EOs needed more than 80 µL/mL to reach such a decline in viability. However, apart from mint, all EOs produced 0% to 10% viability when concentrations were increased to 100 µL/mL.

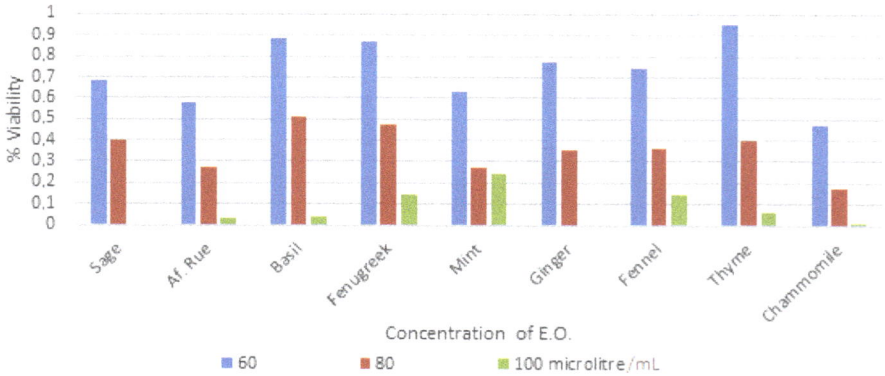

(a) Viability test of by trypan blue on HT-29 (MS) cell lines

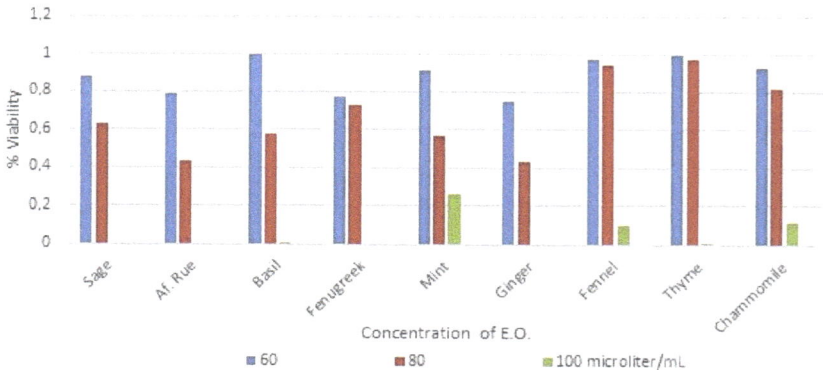

(b) Viability test of by trypan blue on HT-29 A (19) cell lines

Figure 1. Viability percentages of: (**a**) HT29-19(A) non-muco secreting and (**b**) HT29-muco secreting (MS) cell lines treated for 48 h with EOs.

Photos of ginger oil effect on cells at different time intervals are shown in Figure 2a–c.

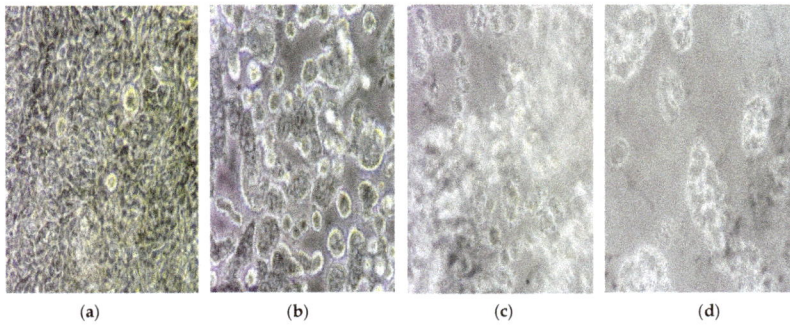

(a)	(b)	(c)	(d)

Figure 2. Effect of ginger oil on the HT-29 (MS) cell line as observed under the microscope. × 400 (**a**), represents cells at time 0 min; (**b–d**) cell at 30 min intervals after ginger oil addition.

3.3. MTT Assay

The MTT cytotoxicity test for both cell lines is shown in Figure 3a,b. IC_{50} for EOs using HT-29 (MS) has revealed that ginger was the lowest in concentration to achieve IC_{50} followed by African rue and sage, with 40, 48 and 53 μL/mL respectively. Whereas, the rest of EOs showed IC_{50} at contents around 80 μL/mL. In the HT-29 19(A) cells, the same trend was obtained, in which ginger got the lowest concentration (60 μL/mL) then thyme was the highest with 77 μL/mL.

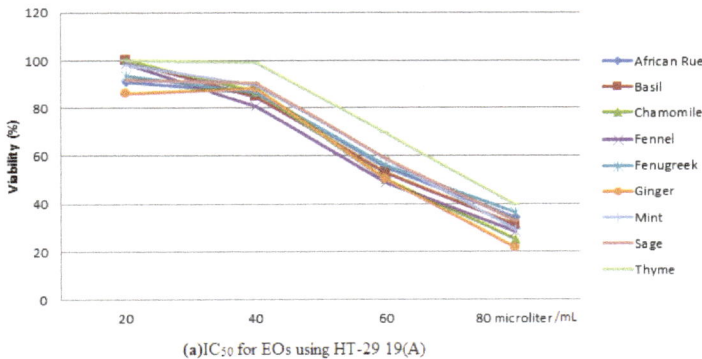

(a)IC_{50} for EOs using HT-29 19(A)

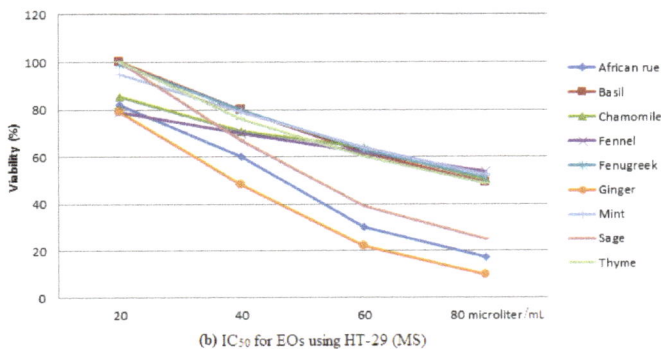

(b) IC_{50} for EOs using HT-29 (MS)

Figure 3. MTT assay using cell lines treated with EOs for 48 h: (**a**) IC_{50} on HT-29 19(A); (**b**) IC_{50} on HT-29 (MS).

3.4. DPPH Radical Scavenging

The reduction ability of DPPH radicals' formation was determined by the decrease in the absorbance at 517 nm induced by antioxidants. DPPH is a stable free radical and accepts an electron (hydrogen radical) to become a stable diamagnetic molecule. A DPPH assay revealed that all commercial EOs assayed in this study have got a very weak or no scavenging capacity compared with the control. These results may be a result of the low quality control of the production or the handling of these EOs products.

Scavenging activity was equivalent to ≤20 µg/mL quercetin, which was the lowest concentration used in the experiment.

3.5. Apoptosis

Ginger oil failed to show an ability to induce apoptosis within the time frame of this experiment. On the other side, caspase-3 activity has not been detected. The same was found for the rest of the EOs. This may be justified by the change in quality of the EOs composition due to many factors including the oxidation, adulteration, or aging [20,21]. As for the S-1 sample, the total amount was determined.

4. Discussion

As it can be noticed from the trypan blue experiment results, most of the EOs have been shown to have a similar trend to inhibit 50% growth (IC$_{50}$) at the content of 80 µL/mL. Indeed, chamomile was very effective when used on HT-29 (MS), whereas, ginger and African rue showed superior effect in comparison with other EOs on HT-29 19(A) cells.

From the latest studies, ginger constituents were reported to have a vital effect in the control of tumor development through up-regulation of the tumor suppressor gene, induction of apoptosis and inactivation of VEGF pathways. For instance, 6-gingerol was found to have a role in the suppression of the hyper-proliferation, transformation, and inflammatory routes that take part in numerous steps of carcinogenesis, angiogenesis and metastasis; in addition, it acts in the initiation of apoptosis in the prostate cancer cell line via inhibition of cell invasion reduction of matrix metalloproteinase-9 expression. Also, 6-gingerol stimulates apoptosis through up-regulation of NAG-1 and G1 cell cycle arrest through down-regulation of cyclin D1 [22]. Besides, other abundant terpenoids also have been found to be present in the ginger like, neral, geranial, zingerberene, camphene, and other oxygenated monoterpenes [23] which may exert a synergistic anticancer activity.

Otherwise, *Peganum harmala* is traditionally used to treat many diseases including cancer. Recent studies show that the alkaloids of *Peganum harmala* are cytotoxic to several tumor cell lines in vitro and have an antitumor effect in a tumor model in vivo. Harmine, a major identified indole alkaloid in the African rue and vasicinone, were the most potent components in inhibiting cell growth and as an antiproliferating agent [24,25]. The active principle at a dose of 50 mg/kg given orally to mice for 40 days was found to have significant anti-tumoral activity [26].

The only difference between both cell lines was the ability of cells to secrete mucus. The negative effect of chamomile, in the case of HT-29 19 (A) cells, is not clear. Mucus in the gut plays a major role in protecting the gut linen from foreign (bio)chemicals. In vitro, a lack of secreting mucus may induce other protective mechanisms that enabled HT-29 19(A) to withstand the impact of higher concentration of EOs. However, as soon as this mechanism was damaged, the viability dramatically declined. On the other side, protection, by mucus, from the effect of the EOs in HT-29 (MS) has gradually decreased as the concentrations of the EOs were increasing.

Scavenging ability of antioxidants decreases by several factors, such as direct light exposure, storage temperature and processing (time needed in open air and temperature) [20]. Commercial EOs are treated and stored in a way in which they can lose their antioxidant and other biological properties. Indeed, there are inevitable factors due to oxidation in the extraction process and in the storage bulk scale of essential oil [20]. Moreover, in Palestine, some EOs are displayed on the shelves in transparent containers, and the temperature may exceed 35 °C in summer time. However, the compositional change in the EOs may be unavoidable even at 5 °C. Such bad preservation conditions may prevent the products from retaining their ability as free radical scavengers.

In fact, EOs which possess high levels of unsaturation might be generally unstable due to many factors such as heat, light, hydration and oxidation.

5. Conclusions

From the EOs tested in this study, we noticed that some had potential activities against the cancer cell tested. Interestingly, in this work, chamomile oil showed the lowest IC_{50} at a content of 60 µL/mL in HT-29 (MS) cell lines. In HT-29 19(A) cells, 50% of the viability was obtained when 80 µL/mL of ginger and African rue EOs were used. An MTT assay on HT-29 (MS) cells showed that ginger IC_{50} was the lowest, followed by African rue and sage, with 40, 48 and 53 µL/mL, respectively. On the other hand, ginger had the lowest IC_{50} with 60 µL/mL whilst thyme was the highest with 77 µL/mL in HT-29 19(A) cells. However, the used commercial EOs did not show any biological activities in the antioxidant and caspase-3 assays.

Factors such as processing, handling, and storage conditions may be responsible for the faintness in the biological and pharmacological properties of the commercial EOs, which originally possess significant biological activities, suggesting that more investigation on commercial Eos is required before recommending their use to the public.

Acknowledgments: The authors acknowledge the help of Zamalah and Cooperative Bank, Palestine for funding through research project.

Author Contributions: The list authors contributed to this work as follows: M.A.A.-T. and B.R. conceived and designed the experiments; M.A.A.-T. and I.M.A.-R. performed research and analyzed the data and wrote the paper. B.R., I.M.A.-R. polished the paper. All authors read and approved the final manuscript.

Conflicts of Interest: The authors declare no conflict of interest.

References

1. Lis-Balchin, M. Essential oils and 'aromatherapy': Their modern role in healing. *J. R. Soc. Promot. Health* **1997**, *117*, 324–329. [CrossRef]

2. Alzeer, B.J.; Vummidi, R.; Arafeh, R.; Rimawi, W.; Saleem, H.; Luedtke, N.W. The influence of extraction solvents on the anticancer activities of Palestinian medicinal plants. *J. Med. Plants Res.* **2014**, *8*, 408–415.

3. Christaki, E.; Bonos, E.; Giannenas, I.; Florou-Paneri, P. Aromatic Plants as a Source of Bioactive Compounds. *Agriculture* **2012**, *2*, 228–243. [CrossRef]

4. Bruneton, J. *Pharmacognosy, Phytochemistry, Medicinal Plants*; Technique & Documentation; Lavoisier: Andover, France, 1999.

5. Turek, C.; Stintzing, F.C. Stability of Essential Oils: A Review. *Compr. Rev. Food Sci. Food Saf.* **2013**, *12*, 40–53. [CrossRef]

6. Baser, K.H.C.; Buchbauer, G. *Handbook of Essential Oils: Science, Technology, and Applications*; CRC Press: Boca Raton, FL, USA, 2009.

7. Calo, J.R.; Crandall, P.G.; O'Bryan, C.A.; Ricke, S.C. Essential oils as antimicrobials in food systems—Review. *Food Control* **2015**, *54*, 111–119. [CrossRef]

8. Hyldgaard, M.; Mygind, T.; Meyer, R.L. Essential Oils in Food Preservation: Mode of Action, Synergies, and Interactions with Food Matrix Components. *Front. Microbiol.* **2012**, *3*. [CrossRef] [PubMed]

9. Li, Y.; Fabiano-Tixier, A.S.; Chémat, F. *Essential Oils as Reagents in Green Chemistry*; Springer: Avignon, France, 2014.

10. Lubbe, A.; Verpoorte, R. Cultivation of medicinal and aromatic plants for specialty industrial materials. *Ind. Crops Prod.* **2011**, *34*, 785–801. [CrossRef]

11. Reuter, S.; Gupta, S.C.; Chaturvedi, M.M.; Aggarwal, B.B. Oxidative stress, inflammation, and cancer: How are they linked? *Free Radic. Biol. Med.* **2010**, *49*, 1603–1616. [CrossRef] [PubMed]

12. Moylan, J.S.; Reid, M.B. Oxidative stress, chronic disease, and muscle wasting. *Muscle Nerve* **2007**, *35*, 411–429. [CrossRef] [PubMed]
13. Tantamango-Bartley, Y.; Jaceldo-Siegl, K.; Fan, J.; Fraser, G. Vegetarian Diets and the Incidence of Cancer in a Low-risk Population. *Cancer Epidemiol. Biomark. Prev.* **2013**, *22*, 286–294. [CrossRef] [PubMed]
14. Namvar, F.; Rahman, H.S.; Mohamad, R.; Baharara, J.; Mahdavi, M.; Amini, E.; Chartrand, M.S.; Yeap, S.K. Cytotoxic effect of magnetic iron oxide nanoparticles synthesized via seaweed aqueous extract. *Int. J. Nanomed.* **2014**, *9*, 2479–2488. [CrossRef] [PubMed]
15. Bayala, B.; Bassole, I.H.; Scifo, R.; Gnoula, C.; Morel, L.; Lobaccaro, J.-M.A.; Simpore, J. Anticancer activity of essential oils and their chemical components—A review. *Am. J. Cancer Res.* **2014**, *4*, 591–607. [PubMed]
16. Bayala, B.; Bassole, I.H.; Gnoula, C.; Nebie, R.; Yonli, A.; Morel, L.; Figueredo, G.; Nikiema, J.B.; Lobaccaro, J.M.; Simpore, J. Chemical Composition, Antioxidant, Anti-Inflammatory and Anti-Proliferative Activities of Essential Oils of Plants from Burkina Faso. *PLoS ONE* **2014**, *9*. [CrossRef] [PubMed]
17. Sak, K. Cytotoxicity of dietary flavonoids on different human cancer types. *Int. J. Pharmacogn.* **2014**, *8*, 122–146. [CrossRef] [PubMed]
18. Gordaliza, M. Natural products as leads to anticancer drugs. *Clin. Transl. Oncol.* **2007**, *9*, 767–776. [CrossRef] [PubMed]
19. Nóbrega de Almeida, R.; Agra, M.D.F.; Souto Maior, F.N.; Pergentino de Sousa, D. Essential oils and their constituents: Anticonvulsant activity. *Molecules* **2011**, *16*, 2726–2742. [CrossRef] [PubMed]
20. Sawamura, M.; Son, U.-S.; Choi, H.-S.; Kim, M.-S.L.; Fears, M.; Phi, N.T.L.; Kumagai, C. Compositional changes in commercial lemon essential oil for aromatherapy. *Int. J. Aromather.* **2004**, *14*, 27–36. [CrossRef]
21. Wabner, D. The peroxide value—A new tool for the quality control of essential oils. *Int. J. Aromather.* **2002**, *12*, 216–218. [CrossRef]
22. Molyneux, P. The use of the stable free radical diphenylpicrylhydrazyl (DPPH) for estimating antioxidant activity. *Songklanakarin J. Sci. Technol.* **2004**, *26*, 211–219.
23. Chagonda, L.S.; Chalchat, J.-C. Essential oil Composition of *Zingiber officinale* Roscoe from Eastern Zimbabwe. *J. Essent. Oil Bear. Plants* **2016**, *19*, 510–515. [CrossRef]
24. Lamchouri, F.; Zemzami, M.; Jossang, A.; Abdellatif, A.; Israili, Z.H.; Lyoussi, B. Cytotoxicity of alkaloids isolated from Peganum harmala seeds. *Pak. J. Pharm. Sci.* **2013**, *26*, 699–706. [PubMed]
25. Aihetasham, A.; Umer, M.; Akhtar, M.S.; Din, M.I.; Rasib, K.Z. Bioactivity of medicinal plants *Mentha arvensis* and *Peganum harmala* extracts against *Heterotermes indicola* (Wasmann) (Isoptera). *Int. J. Biosci.* **2015**, *7*, 116–126.
26. Lamchouri, F.; Settaf, A.; Cherrah, Y.; Zemzami, M.; Lyoussi, B.; Zaid, A.; Atif, N.; Hassar, M. Antitumour principles from *Peganum harmala* seeds. *Therapie* **1999**, *54*, 753–758. [PubMed]

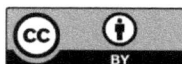

medicines

MDPI

Article

Methanol Extract from *Anogeissus leiocarpus* (DC) Guill. et Perr. (Combretaceae) Stem Bark Quenches the Quorum Sensing of *Pseudomonas aeruginosa* PAO1

Vincent Ouedraogo and Martin Kiendrebeogo *

Laboratoire de Biochimie & Chimie Appliquées, Université Ouaga 1 Pr. Joseph KI-ZERBO,
Ouagadougou, 03 BP 7021, Burkina Faso; vicenteoued@gmail.com
* Correspondence: martinkiendrebeogo@yahoo.co.uk; Tel.: +226-70-608-590

Academic Editor: James D. Adams
Received: 27 August 2016; Accepted: 29 September 2016; Published: 6 October 2016

Abstract: Background: Due to its extensive arsenal of virulence factors and inherent resistance to antibiotics, *Pseudomonas aeruginosa* is a threat particularly in immunocompromised patients. Considering the central role of quorum sensing in the production of virulence factors, inhibition of bacterial communication mechanism constitute an opportunity to attenuate pathogenicity of bacteria resistant to available antibiotics. Our study aimed to assess the anti-quorum sensing activity of *Anogeissus leiocarpus*, traditionally used in Burkina Faso, for the treatment of infected burn wounds. **Methods:** Investigations were carried out on methanol extract from *A. leiocarpus* stem bark. The reporter strains *Chromobacterium violaceum* CV026 and *P. aeruginosa* PAO1 derivatives were used to evidence any interference with the bacterial quorum sensing and expression of related genes. *P. aeruginosa* PAO1 was used to measure the impact on pyocyanin production. **Results:** At a sub-inhibitory concentration (100 µg/mL), *A. leiocarpus* methanol extract quenched the quorum sensing mechanism of *P. aeruginosa* PAO1 by down-streaming the *rhlR* gene, with a subsequent reduction of pyocyanin production. Moreover, the antioxidant polyphenols evidenced are able to reduce the oxidative stress induced by pyocyanin. **Conclusion:** The antioxidant and anti-quorum sensing activities of *A. leiocarpus* stem bark could justify its traditional use in the treatment of infected burn wounds.

Keywords: *Anogeissus leiocarpus*; *Chromobacterium violaceum* CV026; *Pseudomonas aeruginosa* PAO1; pyocyanin; quorum sensing

---

1. Introduction

Pseudomonas aeruginosa infections are common following burn injuries [1] and often present as wound infections [2]. Due to its extensive arsenal of virulence factors and inherent resistance to several antibiotics, approximately 80% of burn patients infected with *P. aeruginosa* die of septicaemia [3]. Production of virulence factors by *P. aeruginosa* is under the control of a cell-to-cell communication system termed quorum sensing (QS), which is a mechanism used by many bacteria to detect their critical cell numbers through the release and perception of small diffusible signal molecules called auto inducers, in order to coordinate a common behavior [4–6].

In *P. aeruginosa*, two QS systems (lasI/lasR and rhlI/RhlR) drive the production (by the synthetases LasI and RhlI) and the perception (by the transcription factors LasR and RhlR) of the auto inducers acyl homoserine lactones (AHL)—*N*-(3-oxododecanoyl)-L-homoserine lactone (3-oxo-C12-HSL) and *N*-butanoyl-L-homoserine lactone (C4-HSL), respectively [4,5,7,8]. A third

QS system, based on quinolone signals, links and interacts in an intricate way with the lasI/lasR and rhlI/RhlR quorum-sensing systems [9–12].

Following injuries, inflammation process (representing a non-specific immune response to chemical or biological aggression) takes place in order to pathogen elimination and tissue injury reparation [13–15].

Inflammatory reactions start with the release of inflammatory mediators (e.g., cytokines, endotoxins, prostaglandins, leukotrienes, and histamine) as well as reactive oxygen species (ROS) by injured cells.

In non-pathogenic conditions, cells are normally able to defend themselves against ROS damage through the use of endogen enzymatic and non-enzymatic antioxidants agents. Since *P. aeruginosa* infection during a burn wound dramatically boosts the level of ROS, antioxidant defense systems of cells are overpassed, resulting in oxidative stress with significant damage to cell structures [16,17].

In the ongoing struggle against bacterial infection, antibiotics are commonly used to kill pathogenic bacteria. However, bacteria increasingly exhibit resistance against available antimicrobial drugs [18,19]. To cope with these limitations, the alternative approach consisting in attenuating the expression of bacterial virulence factor without affecting their viability by using anti-QS agents has become a rational preventive strategy [20,21].

In Burkina Faso, more than 80% of the population relies on traditional practices and medicinal plants to treat various diseases [22]. Some medicinal plants have been reported to present anti-inflammatory activity and wound healing effects without any antibacterial activity [22,23], which suggests a non-antimicrobial modulation of virulence factors.

In this study, *Anogeissus leiocarpus* (DC) Guill. & Perr. (Combretaceae), which is traditionally involved in Burkina Faso for the treatment of infected burn wounds [22], was investigated for its ability to reduce the production of pyocyanin, one of the QS-controlled virulence factors produced by *P. aeruginosa*, and to interfere with the bacterial QS system. Total polyphenol and flavonoid content as well as the antioxidant potentiality of this medicinal plant were also assessed.

2. Materials and Methods

2.1. Bacterial Strains, Plasmids, and Culture Conditions

Chromobacterium violaceum CV026, *Pseudomonas aeruginosa* PAO1, and its derivatives (Table S1) harboring plasmids pPCS1001 (P_{lasR}-*lacZ* transcriptional fusion), pβ03 (P_{lasI}-*lacZ* transcriptional fusion), pPCS1002 (P_{rhlR}-*lacZ* transcriptional fusion), pLPR1 (P_{rhlI}-*lacZ* transcriptional fusion), pTB4124 (P_{acAe}-*lacZ* transcriptional fusion) and pβ02 (P_{rhlA}-*lacZ* transcriptional fusion) were provided from the Laboratoire de Biotechnologie Vegetale (Université Libre de Bruxelles, Gosselies, Belgium). *P. aeruginosa* PAO1 (37 °C, agitation 175 rpm) and *C. violaceum* CV026 (30 °C, agitation 175 rpm) were grown in LB broth. *P. aeruginosa* PAO1 derivatives strains were grown (37 °C, agitation 175 rpm) in LB-MOPS broth (50 mM, pH 7) supplemented with carbenicillin (300 µg/mL).

2.2. Plant Material Collection and Extraction

Stem bark of *Anogeissus leiocarpus* (DC) Guill. et Perr. (Combretaceae) was collected in August 2014 at Gampela (25 km, east of Ouagadougou, Burkina Faso). Botanical identity was assessed by Dr. Amade Ouedraogo from the Laboratoire de Biologie et Ecologie Vegetale (Université Ouaga 1 Pr. Joseph Ki-Zerbo, Ouagadougou, Burkina Faso) where a voucher specimen (ID: 16883) was deposited. Plant material was dried at room temperature, ground into fine powder, and stored in an airtight bag until use.

Powdered plant material (100 g) was defatted with petroleum ether (500 mL) in a soxhlet extractor (Wheaton industries Inc., Millvile, NJ, USA) and soaked (24 h, 25 °C, continuous stirring) in methanol. Extract was filtrated, concentrated in a vacuum evaporator (Büchi Labortechnik AG, Postfach, Flawil, Switzerland) and dried to obtain 14.4 g of plant extract. Plant extract (100 mg/mL) was dissolve either in methanol for phytochemical purpose or in dimethyl sulfoxide (DMSO) for testing on bacterial strains. Test samples were stored at 4 °C until use.

2.3. Total Polyphenol and Flavonoid Content Determination

Total polyphenol was determined according to the colorimetric method of Folin–Ciocalteu [24]. Plant extract (25 μL, 100 μg/mL in methanol) was mixed with Folin–Ciocalteu Reagent (125 μL, 0.2 N) and, 5 min later, with sodium bicarbonate (100 μL, 75 g/L). After incubation (1 h, room temperature), absorbance was measured at 760 nm against a methanol blank. Gallic acid (0–100 mg/L) was used to generate a standard calibration curve ($Y = 0.005X + 0.00968$; $R^2 = 0.99$), and total polyphenol content was expressed as mg gallic acid equivalent to 100 mg of plant extract (mg GAE/100 mg).

Total flavonoid was estimated according to the Dowd method [24]. Plant extract (75 μL, 100 μg/mL in methanol) was mixed with aluminium trichloride (75 μL, 2% in methanol). Absorbance was subsequently read at 415 nm after incubation (10 min, room temperature) against a methanol blank. Quercetin (0–100 mg/L) was used to plot a standard calibration curve ($Y = 0.02891X + 0.0036$; $R^2 = 0.99$), and total flavonoid content was expressed as mg of quercetin equivalent to 100 mg of plant extract (mg QE/100 mg).

2.4. Antioxidant Assays

Antioxidant activity was measured through 2,2-diphenyl-1-picrylhydrazyl (DPPH) and ferric reducing antioxidant power (FRAP) assays as previously described [24].

For the DPPH assay, freshly prepared DPPH solution (200 μL, 0.02 mg/mL in methanol) was mixed with plant extract (100 μL, 100 to 0.39 μg/mL in methanol). The mixture was subsequently shacked and incubated (15 min in darkness, room temperature), and absorbance was measured at 517 nm against a methanol blank. DPPH radical scavenging activities were plotted against sample concentrations, and the result was expressed as a sample concentration scavenging 50% of DPPH radicals (IC50). Quercetin was used as positive controls.

For FRAP testing, plant extract (100 μL, 100 μg/mL in methanol) was mixed with a phosphate buffer (250 μL, 0.2 M, pH 6.6) and a potassium hexacyanoferrate solution (250 μL, 1% in water). After incubation (30 min, 50 °C), trichloroacetic acid (250, 10% in water) was added, and the mixture centrifuged ($2000 \times g$ for 10 min). The supernatant (125 μL) was mixed with water (125 μL) and a fresh FeCl$_3$ solution (25 μL, 0.1% in water) to read absorbance at 700 nm. Ascorbic acid was used to plot a calibration curve ($R^2 = 0.99$). Reducing power was expressed as μM ascorbic acid equivalent per gram of plant extract (μM AAE/g). Quercetin was used as positive controls.

2.5. Determination of MIC and MBC

MIC (minimum inhibitory concentration) values on *P. aeruginosa* PAO1 and *C. violaceum* CV026 were determined according to the micro dilution method, using *p*-iodonitrotetrazolium (INT) as an indicator of bacterial growth [25]. In brief, an overnight bacterial culture was diluted with LB broth to obtain a starting inoculum (109 CFU/mL). Inoculum (180 μL) was added to serial dilutions of test extract (20 μL; 50 to 0.39 mg/mL in DMSO 10%) to obtain a final concentration range of 5 mg/mL to 0.039 mg/mL. Mixtures were incubated for 18 h (37 °C, 175 rpm agitation). After 18 h of incubation, 50 μL of INT (0.2 mg/mL) was added to each well, and the microplate was further incubated (37 °C, 30 min). Bacterial growth was indicated by a red color within the microplate wells (Greiner Bio-One GmbH, Frieckenhausen, Germany).

To determine the MBC, aliquots of 20 μL from all dilutions not showing any bacterial growth were spread onto LB agar plates and incubated (37 °C, 24 h). The minimum concentration for which there is no visible growth on agar plate was recorded as MBC [26].

2.6. Quantitative Analysis of Pyocyanin Production in P. aeruginosa PAO1

Inhibition of pyocyanin production was assessed according to previously described procedures [27]. *P. aeruginosa* PAO1 was grown (18 h in LB broth, 37 °C, 175 rpm agitation), and cells were washed twice in fresh LB medium. In 18 culture tubes, appropriately diluted PAO1 cell suspension (250 μL) was added to the LB medium (4.7 mL, starting OD600nm ranged between 0.02 and 0.03) and supplemented with plant extract (50 μL, 10 mg/mL in DMSO) or DMSO. At periodic time intervals (3 h), tubes (*n* = 3) were sampled to assess bacterial growth (ufc/mL) and pyocyanin content.

From each tube, 100 μL of bacterial culture were removed and diluted in LB broth to be plated onto LB agar and incubated (24 h, 37 °C) for colony counting, while 200 μL of bacterial culture was used to determine optical density at 600 nm. Remaining bacterial culture was centrifuged (7000 rpm, 10 min, 24 °C) to obtain culture supernatant. Pyocyanin was extracted from the supernatant (4 mL) with chloroform (2 mL) and re-extracted from chloroform with 0.2 M HCl (1 mL). Optical density reading at 380 nm allows pyocyanin determination.

2.7. Quantitative Analysis of Violacein Production in C. violaceum CV026

Inhibition of violacein production in *C. violaceum* CV026 was tested according to [27]. Violacein production was induced in *C. violaceum* CV026 by adding exogenous *N*-hexanoyl-L-homoserine lactone (HHL; Sigma-Aldrich Chemie GmbH, Darmstadt, Germany).

An appropriately diluted overnight culture of *C. violaceum* CV026 (200 μL) was incubated (30 °C, 48 h, 175 rpm agitation) in 18 culture tubes containing LB broth (4.7 mL) supplemented with HHL (50 μL, 10 mM in DMSO) and plant extract (50 μL, 10 mg/mL in DMSO) or DMSO. At periodic time intervals (6 h), tubes (*n* = 3) were sampled to assess bacterial growth (ufc/mL and OD600 nm) and pyocyanin content, while violacein was quantified after 48 h growth.

From each tube, bacterial culture (1 mL) was centrifuged (7000 rpm, 10 min) and DMSO (1 mL) was added to the pellet. The solution was vortexed to dissolve violacein, and cell debris was discarded by centrifugation (7000 rpm, 10 min). Violacein content in supernatant was measured by the absorbance at 585 nm.

2.8. β-Galactosidase Assay

β-Galactosidase measurements were performed as previously described [27]. After growth in liquid LB-MOPS-Carbenicillin (37 °C with 175 rpm agitation) for 18 h, PAO1 reporter strains harboring plasmids (Table S1) were washed twice in fresh LB medium and resuspended in fresh liquid LB-MOPS-Carbenicillin. PAO1 reporter strains inoculums (50 μL) were incubated (37 °C with 175 rpm agitation) for 8 or 18 h in 1 mL of LB-MOPS-Carbenicillin (initial OD600 nm of culture comprised between 0.020 and 0.025) supplemented with 10 μL of plant extracts (100 μg/mL final concentration) or 10 μL of DMSO. After incubation, bacterial density was assessed by spectrophotometry (OD600 nm), and the sample used for cell growth assessment was used to perform the β-galactosidase assay with O-nitrophenyl-β-D-galactopyranoside as described elsewhere [28].

2.9. Statistical Analysis

All experiments were performed in triplicate (independent assays), and data were expressed as mean ± SD. Data analysis was performed via analysis of variance (one-way ANOVA or two-way ANOVA) followed by a Tukey or Bonferonni test, using GraphPad Prism software (version 5.00 for window, GraphPad Software, San Diego, CA, USA) *p* value ≤ 0.05 was considered significant.

3. Results

3.1. Antioxidant Activity, Total Polyphenol, and Flavovoid Content

Total polyphenol and total flavonoid were quantified from methanol extract of *A. leiocarpus* stem bark together with its antioxidant capacity through radicals DPPH scavenging activity and ferric reducing power, and each antioxidant assay involved a different antioxidant mechanism. The amount of total polyphenol was particularly high (82.62 ± 3.16 mg GAE/100 mg) in addition to a low content of total flavonoid (15.14 ± 0. 39 mg QE/100 mg). As shown, an interesting antioxidant potential was found. *A. leiocarpus* exhibits the same DPPH radical scavenging activity (1.82 ± 0.07 µg/mL) as quercetin (1.40 ± 0.15 µg/mL), while its ferric-reducing power (4.29 ± 0.19 µM AAE/g) was only two-fold lower than that of our antioxidant reference (7.66 ± 0.39 µM AAE/g).

3.2. Inhibition of Pyocianin Production

The MIC (1.25 mg/mL) and MBC (>5.00 mg/mL) values evaluated allow for the selection of a sub-inhibitory concentration for the bioassay on *P. aeruginosa* PAO1. Methanol extract from *A. leiocarpus* stem bark (100 µg/mL) was incubated for 18 h in *P. aeruginosa* PAO1 culture to access its capacity to interfere with the production of pyocyanin, a QS-dependent extracellular virulence factor of the bacteria. As shown, methanol extract from *A. leiocarpus* (100 µg/mL final concentration) significantly impact ($p < 0.05$) in a kinetic way the production of pyocyanin (Figure 1a) without any effect on bacterial kinetic growth (Figure 1b). Hence, the reduction of pyocyanin production recorded within 18 h was not the consequence of any bactericidal or bacteriostatic effect but probably the effect of some interference with the QS mechanism of *P. aeruginosa* PAO1, controlling the production of pyocyanin.

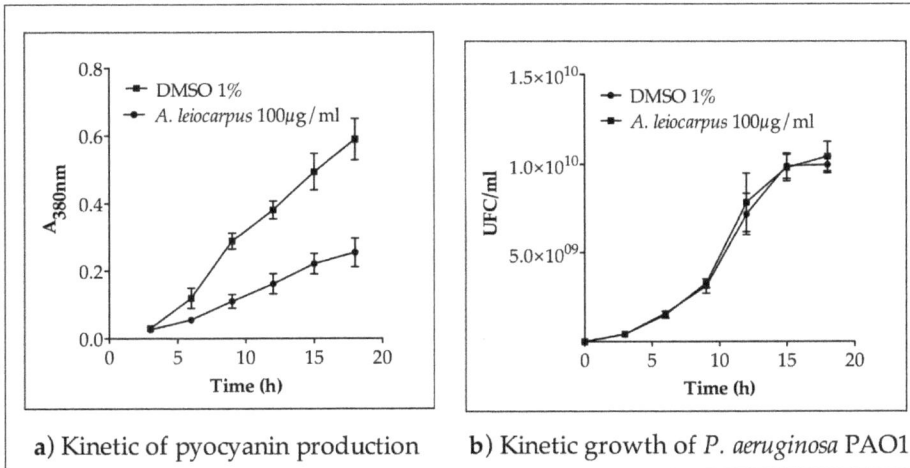

a) Kinetic of pyocyanin production   b) Kinetic growth of *P. aeruginosa* PAO1

Figure 1. Methanol extract from *A. leiocarpus* reduce pyocyanin production in *P. aeruginosa* PAO1. (**a**) *A. leiocarpus* extract (100 µg/mL) significantly reduced ($p > 0.05$) pyocyanin production within 18 h compared to DMSO used as control; (**b**) *A. leiocarpus* extract (100 µg/mL) did not exhibit a significant effect on *P. aeruginosa* PAO1 kinetic growth within 18 h. Dimethyl sulfoxide (DMSO) was used as negative control. *P. aeruginosa* PAO1 was grown (37 °C, 175 rpm agitation) in the LB broth. Mean values ± SD of triplicate independent experiments are shown.

3.3. Anti-Quorum Sensing Activity

To assess the ability of the methanol extract from *A leiocarpus* stem bark to interfere with the quorum sensing mechanism, the reporter strain *C. violaceum* CV026, deficient in the homoserine-lactone synthase gene *cviI*, was used. This strain is unable to produce quorum sensing auto inducers (homoserine-lactones) by itself, nor therefore the QS-related violacein, without an external supply of homoserine-lactone. The MIC (0.62 mg/mL) and MBC (2.50 mg/mL) values evaluated allow for the selection of a sub-inhibitory concentration for the bioassay on *C. violaceum* CV026. Methanol extract from *A. leiocarpus* (100 μg/mL final concentration) reduced violacein production by up to 50% (Figure 2a) without any effect on bacterial kinetic growth (Figure 2b). Therefore, the reduction of violacein production observed was not due to any bactericidal or bacteriostatic effect, but to a quenching of the QS system of the bacteria. When extract was added to *C. violaceum* CV026 growth medium without a HHL supply, violacein was not produced, indicating that *A. leiocarpus* extract do not contain mimic HHL compound (data not shown).

In order to evidence any interference with the expression of quorum sensing (QS) genes of *P. aeruginosa* PAO1, we focused on the transcriptional level after 18 h of incubation. Therefore, the expression of the HHL synthetases genes (*lasI* and *rhlI*), the QS regulator genes (*lasR* and *rhlR*), and the virulence factor QS-controlled genes (*lasB* and *rhlA*) were evaluated. As shown (Figure 3), methanol extract of *A. leiocarpus* stem bark did not significantly affect ($p < 0.05$) the transcription level of the quorum sensing *lasI*, *lasR*, and *rhlI* genes, while expression of *rhlR* was significantly ($p < 0.05$) downstreamed.

To determine whether the drop in β-galactosidase activity recorded was not due to an effect on the transcription/translation mechanisms, nor to an inhibition of the enzyme (β-galactosidase), a *P. aeruginosa* PAO1 strain harboring the aceA-lacZ fusion (*aceA* gene encoding for isocitrate lyase) was tested. As shown, *A. leiocarpus* extract had no effect on the transcription of the *aceA* gene, demonstrating that it affects the expression of QS-related genes without interfering with the entire transcription machinery of *P. aeruginosa* PAO1. Hence, *A. leiocarpus* methanol extract clearly exhibited anti-QS activity on *P. aeruginosa* PAO1.

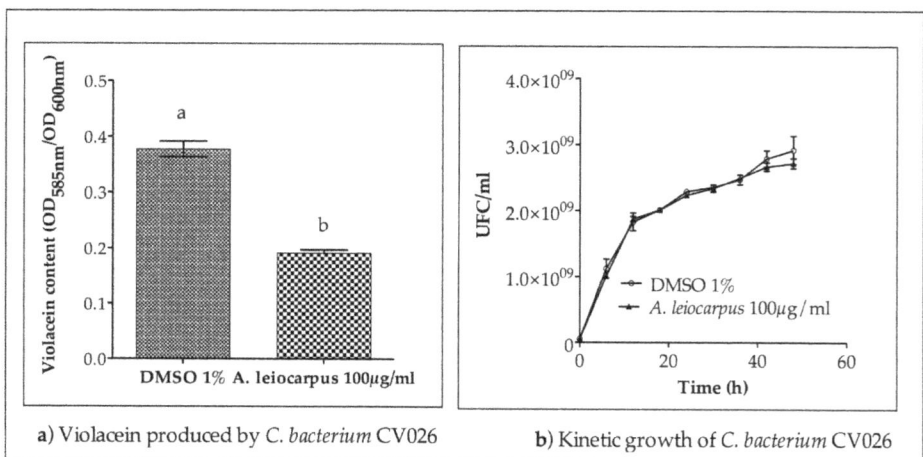

a) Violacein produced by *C. bacterium* CV026   b) Kinetic growth of *C. bacterium* CV026

Figure 2. Anti-quorum sensing (QS) activity of methanol extract from *A. leiocarpus*. (**a**) *A. leiocarpus* extract (100 μg/mL) significantly reduces ($p > 0.05$) violacein production by *C. violaceum* CV026 within 48 h (**b**) *A. leiocarpus* extract (100 μg/mL) did not exhibit a significant effect of on *C. violaceum* CV026 kinetic growth within 48 h. Dimethyl sulfoxide (DMSO) was used as a negative control. *C. violaceum* CV026 was grown (30 °C, 175 rpm agitation) in LB broth supplemented with HHL (10 μM in DMSO). Mean values of triplicate independent experiments and SD are shown. Data with different letters in superscript are significantly different ($p > 0.05$).

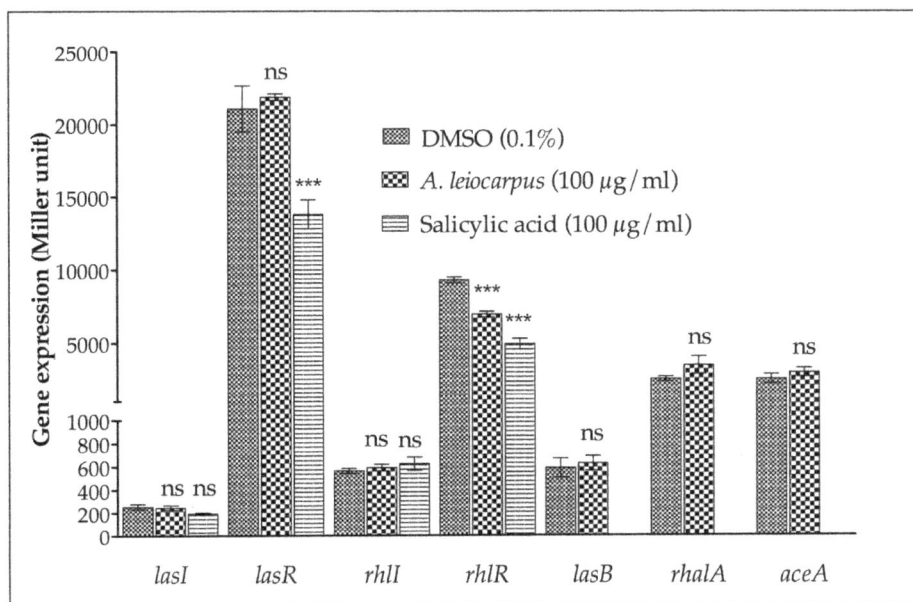

Figure 3. Effect of *A. leiocarpus* extract on the transcription level of *lasRI* and *rhlRI* QS genes. Data are expressed as mean ± SD of 3 independent essays. Dimethyl sulfoxide (DMSO) was used as negative control. Salicylic acid was used as positive control. *** Significantly different compared with DMSO treatment ($p < 0.05$). ns: not significantly different compared to DMSO treatment. Gene expression was measured as the β-galactosidase activity of the *lacZ* gene fusions and expressed in Miller units. Expression of the *aceA* gene is used as a quorum-sensing independent control. *P. aeruginosa* PAO1 strains were grown.

4. Discussion

Our in vitro investigations show that methanol extract from *A. leiocarpus* stem bark exhibits promising antioxidant capacity along with anti-QS activity with a subsequent reduction of pyocyanin production. Since *phz*, the biosynthesis genes of pyocyanin, is under the control of *las* and *rhl* QS systems [29,30], the observed decrease in pyocyanin production is related to the downstreaming of the QS regulator gene *rhlR*.

P. aeruginosa PAO1 QS systems *las* and *rhl* seems to be important for a successful infection in burn wounds, as the virulence of PAO1 mutants defective in either *lasI*, *lasR*, or *rhlI* is reduced [31]. Consistent with this, the inability of QS-deficient strains to induce a successful infection was proposed to be linked with a decreased production of virulence factors such as pyocyanin among other virulence factors, and the most significant virulence reduction was detected with the mutant defective in both *lasI* and *rhlI* [31]. Hence, the anti-QS demonstrated might explain the traditional usage of *A. leiocarpus* stem bark to treat infected burn wounds.

Within the Combretaceae family, to which belongs *A. leiocarpus*, anti-QS medicinal plants have been previously reported. *Bucida buceras*, *Combretum albiflorum*, and *Conocarpus erectus* quench the QS mechanism of *P. aeruginosa* PAO1 with a subsequent inhibition of the bacteria virulence factors [27,32]. Polyphenols and flavonoids are also known for their anti-QS potentiality. The flavonoids catechin, isolated from *Combretum albiflorum* and naringenin have been reported to inhibit QS-regulated virulence factors expression in *P. aeruginosa* and thought to possibly interfere with the perception of the native AHL by LasR and RhlR [27,33]. Epigallocatechin gallate, tannic acid, and ellagic acid also demonstrated their anti-QS potential against *Pseudomonas putida* [34]. Vescalagin and castalagin, two ellagitannins isolated from *Conocarpus erectus*, decrease AHL production, QS gene expression and elastases production [35]. The anti-QS activity and related reduction of pyocyanin production observed within our study might be due to castalagin, since it has been previously isolated from the stem bark of *A. leiocarpus* [36]. Furthermore, 3,3′,4′-tri-*O*-methylflavellagic acid, 3,3′-di-*O*-methylellagic acid, and 3,4,3′-tri-*O*-methylflavellagic acid-4′-β-D-glucoside, three ellagic acid derivatives isolated from *A. leiocarpus* stem bark [37], might contribute to the anti-QS bioactivity we demonstrated.

Among several virulence factors produced by *P. aeruginosa*, pyocyanin is known to be involved in cell host degradation and the production of ROS [38,39]. Pyocyanin alters the redox cycle involved in cellular respiration and increases the oxidative stress on host cells [1]. The mechanism by which pyocyanin causes cell cycle arrest is related to its redox (oxidation–reduction) properties, and its ability to reduce molecular oxygen into reactive oxygen species induces low-level, yet persistent, oxidative stress [40,41]. Thus, pyocyanin is able to delay cicatrization and might also lead to chronic inflammation in wound and burn injuries infected by *P. aeruginosa*. Polyphenols and flavonoids responsible for the antioxidant activity of *A. leiocarpus* could therefore contribute to the reduction of the oxidative stress caused by pyocyanin and thus reduce inflammatory intensity independently of pyocyanin reduction, a benefit for wound healing.

Taken together, anti-QS and antioxidant activities of *A. leiocarpus* could contribute to an explanation of its wound-healing benefit. The antioxidant activities could represent a preventive action to minimize ROS due to inflammation but also counterbalance the high level production of ROS when burn injuries are infected by opportunistic pathogens. Additionally, the anti-QS activity also preserves a minimal ROS level as it reduces virulence factor production such as pyocyanin, and more importantly reduce the abilities of pathogens to degrade host tissue and to resist host immune responses that can maintain inflammation and delay the healing process.

5. Conclusions

Our study demonstrated the antioxidant and anti-QS activities of the methanol extract from *A. leiocarpus* stem bark. Based on bibliographic reports, catalagin and ellagic acid derivatives might be responsible for the anti-QS property demonstrated. These results contribute to the establishment of the traditional use of *A. leiocarpus* stem bark in the management of infected burn wounds on a rational basis. By reducing the production of pyocyanin and related oxidative stress within infected tissues in a QS manner, *A. leiocarpus* stem bark benefits to the healing process of septic injuries.

In future investigations, we will focus on the interference of the anti-QS molecules from *A. leiocarpus* either with the mechanisms of perception or production of homoserine lactones (lasI/lasR, rhlI/rhlR QS systems) or with the quinolone signal (the third QS system) within *P. aeruginosa*.

Supplementary Materials: The following are available online at www.mdpi.com/2305-6320/3/4/26/s1. Table S1: List of plasmids used in this study.

Acknowledgments: The authors are grateful to Prof Mondher EL JAZIRI from the Laboratoire de Biotechnologie Vegetale, Univerté Libre de Bruxelles, Belgium, for providing the bacterial strains used in this study. This research was funded by The World Academy of Science (TWAS) under the research grant 12-044/RG/BIO/AF/AC-G-UNESCO FR: 3240271326.

Author Contributions: M.K. conceived and designed the experiments; V.O. performed the experiments; M.K. and V.O. analyzed the data and wrote the paper; M.K. provided reagents and material through a research grant awarded to him.

Conflicts of Interest: The authors declare no conflict of interest. The founding sponsor had no role in the design of the study; in the collection, analyses, or interpretation of data; in the writing of the manuscript, or in the decision to publish the results.

References

1.   Liu, G.Y.; Nizet, V. Color me bad: Microbial pigments as virulence factors. *Trends Microbiol.* **2009**, *17*, 406–413. [CrossRef] [PubMed]

2. Rumbaugh, K.P.; Griswold, J.A.; Hamood, A.N. The role of quorum sensing in the in vivo virulence of *Pseudomonas aeruginosa*. *Microbes Infect.* **2000**, *2*, 1721–1731. [CrossRef]

3. Richard, P.; le Floch, R.; Chamoux, C.; Pannier, M.; Espaze, E.; Richet, H. *Pseudomonas aeruginosa* outbreak in a burn unit: Role of antimicrobials in the emergence of multiply resistant strains. *J. Infect. Dis.* **1994**, *170*, 377–383. [CrossRef] [PubMed]

4. Greenberg, E.P. Acyl-homosérine lactone quorum sensing in bacteria. *J. Microbiol.* **2000**, *38*, 117–121.

5. Jimenez, P.N.; Koch, G.; Thompson, J.A.; Xavier, K.B.; Cool, R.H.; Quax, W.J. The multiple signaling systems regulating virulence in *Pseudomonas aeruginosa*. *Microbiol. Mol. Biol. Rev.* **2012**, *76*, 46–65. [CrossRef] [PubMed]

6. Parsek, M.R.; Greenberg, E.P. Sociomicrobiology: The connections between quorum sensing and biofilms. *Trends Microbiol.* **2005**, *13*, 27–33. [CrossRef] [PubMed]

7. Pesci, E.C.; Pearson, J.P.; Seed, P.C.; Iglewski, B.H. Regulation of *las* and *rhl* quorum sensing in *Pseudomonas aeruginosa*. *J. Bacteriol.* **1997**, *179*, 3127–3132. [PubMed]

8. Venturi, V. Regulation of quorum sensing in *Pseudomonas*. *FEMS Microbiol. Rev.* **2006**, *30*, 274–291. [CrossRef] [PubMed]

9. Diggle, S.P.; Winzer, K.; Chhabra, S.R.; Worrall, K.E.; Cámara, M.; Williams, P. The *Pseudomonas aeruginosa* quinolone signal molecule overcomes the cell density-dependency of the quorum sensing hierarchy, regulates *rhl*-dependent genes at the onset of stationary phase and can be produced in the absence of LasR. *Mol. Microbiol.* **2003**, *50*, 29–43. [CrossRef] [PubMed]

10. McKnight, S.L.; Iglewski, B.H.; Pesci, E.C. The *Pseudomonas* quinolone signal regulates *rhl* quorum sensing in *Pseudomonas aeruginosa*. *J. Bacteriol.* **2000**, *182*, 2702–2708. [CrossRef] [PubMed]

11. Pesci, E.C.; Milbank, J.B.; Pearson, J.P.; McKnight, S.; Kende, A.S.; Greenberg, E.P.; Iglewski, B.H. Quinolone signaling in the cell-to-cell communication system of *Pseudomonas aeruginosa*. *Proc. Natl. Acad. Sci. USA* **1999**, *96*, 11229–11234. [CrossRef] [PubMed]

12. Wade, D.S.; Calfee, M.W.; Rocha, E.R.; Ling, E.A.; Engstrom, E.; Coleman, J.P.; Pesci, E.C. Regulation of *Pseudomonas* quinolone signal synthesis in *Pseudomonas aeruginosa*. *J. Bacteriol.* **2005**, *187*, 4372–4380. [CrossRef] [PubMed]

13. Gibran, N.S.; Heimbach, D.M. Current status of burn wound pathophysiology. *Clin. Plast. Surg.* **2000**, *27*, 11–22. [PubMed]

14. Farina, J.A., Jr.; Rosique, M.J.; Rosique, R.G. Curbing inflammation in burn patients. *Int. J. Inflamm.* **2013**. [CrossRef] [PubMed]

15. Ward, P.A.; Lentsch, A.B. The acute inflammatory response and its regulation. *Arch. Surg.* **1999**, *134*, 666–669. [CrossRef] [PubMed]

16. Rahman, I.; MacNee, W. Regulation of redox glutathione levels and gene transcription in lung inflammation: Therapeutic approaches. *Free Radic. Biol. Med.* **2000**, *28*, 1405–1420. [CrossRef]

17. Wang, J.; Blanchard, T.G.; Ernst, P.B. *Host Inflammatory Response to Infection in Helicobacter pylori: Physiology and Genetics*; Mobley, H.L.T., Mendz, G.L., Hazell, S.L., Eds.; ASM Press: Washington, DC, USA, 2001.

18. Epps, L.C.; Walker, P.D. Fluoroquinolone consumption and emerging resistance. *US Pharm.* **2006**, *10*, 47–54.

19. English, B.K.; Gaur, A.H. The use and abuse of antibiotics and the development of antibiotic resistance. *Adv. Exp. Med. Biol.* **2010**, *659*, 73–82. [PubMed]

20. Bjarnsholt, T.; Givskov, M. The role of quorum sensing in the pathogenicity of the cunning aggressor *Pseudomonas aeruginosa*. *Anal. Bioanal. Chem.* **2007**, *387*, 409–414. [CrossRef] [PubMed]

21. Hentzer, M.; Givskov, M. Pharmacological inhibition of quorum sensing for the treatment of chronic bacterial infections. *J. Clin. Investig.* **2003**, *112*, 1300–1307. [CrossRef] [PubMed]

22. Nacoulma, O.G. *Plantes Médicinales et Pratiques Médicinales Traditionnelles au Burkina*; Université de Ouagadougou: Ouagadougou, Burkina Faso, 1996. (In French)

23. Agyare, C.; Asase, A.; Lechtenberg, M.; Niehues, M.; Deters, A.; Hensel, A. An ethnopharmacological survey and in vitro confirmation of ethnopharmacological use of medicinal plants used for wound healing in Bosomtwi-Atwima-Kwanwoma area, Ghana. *J. Ethnopharmacol.* **2009**, *125*, 393–403. [CrossRef] [PubMed]

24. Lamien-Meda, A.; Lamien, C.E.; Compaoré, M.M.Y.; Meda, N.T.R.; Kiendrebeogo, M.; Zeba, B.; Millogo, J.F.; Nacoulma, O.G. Polyphenol content and antioxidant activity of fourteen wild edible fruits from Burkina Faso. *Molecules* **2008**, *13*, 581–594. [CrossRef] [PubMed]

25. Eloff, J.N. A sensitive and quick microplate method to determine the minimal inhibitory concentration of plant extracts for bacteria. *Planta Med.* **1998**, *64*, 711–713. [CrossRef] [PubMed]

26. Escalona-Arranz, J.C.; Péres-Roses, R.; Urdaneta-Laffita, I.; Camacho-Pozo, M.I.; Rodríguez-Amado, J.; Licea-Jiménez, I. Antimicrobial activity of extracts from *Tamarindus indica* L. leaves. *Pharmacogn. Mag.* **2010**, *6*, 242–247. [CrossRef] [PubMed]

27. Vandeputte, O.M.; Kiendrebeogo, M.; Rajaonson, S.; Diallo, B.; Mol, A.; El Jaziri, M.; Baucher, M. Identification of catechin as one of the flavonoids from *Combretum albiflorum* bark extract that reduces the production of quorum-sensing-controlled virulence factors in *Pseudomonas aeruginosa* PAO1. *Appl. Environ. Microbiol.* **2010**, *76*, 243–253. [CrossRef] [PubMed]

28. Zhang, X.; Bremer, H. Control of the *Escherichia coli* rrnB P1 promoter strength by ppGpp. *J. Biol. Chem.* **1995**, *270*, 11181–11189. [CrossRef] [PubMed]

29. Pearson, J.P.; Pesci, E.C.; Iglewski, B.H. Roles of *Pseudomonas aeruginosa las* and *rhl* quorum-sensing systems in control of elastase and rhamnolipid biosynthesis genes. *J. Bacteriol.* **1997**, *179*, 5756–5767. [PubMed]

30. Brint, J.; Ohman, D.E. Synthesis of multiple exoproducts in *Pseudomonas aeruginosa* is under the control of RhlR-RhlI, another set of regulators in strain PAO1 with homology to the autoinducer-responsive LuxR-LuxI family. *J. Bacteriol.* **1995**, *177*, 7155–7163. [PubMed]

31. Rumbaugh, K.P.; Griswold, J.A.; Iglewski, B.H.; Hamood, A.N. Contribution of quorum sensing to the virulence of *Pseudomonas aeruginosa* in burn wound infections. *Infect. Immun.* **1999**, *67*, 5854–5862. [PubMed]

32. Adonizio, A.; Kong, K.; Mathee, K. Inhibition of quorum sensing-controlled virulence factor production in *Pseudomonas aeruginosa* by south Florida plant extracts. *Antimicrob. Agents Chemother.* **2008**, *52*, 198–203. [CrossRef] [PubMed]

33. Vandeputte, O.M.; Kiendrebeogo, M.; Rasamiravaka, T.; Stévigny, C.; Duez, P.; Rajaonson, S.; Diallo, B.; Mol, A.; Baucher, M.; El Jaziri, M. The flavanone naringenin reduces the production of quorum sensing-controlled virulence factors in *Pseudomonas aeruginosa* PAO1. *Microbiology* **2011**, *157*, 2120–2132. [CrossRef] [PubMed]

34. Huber, B.; Eberl, L.; Feucht, W.; Polster, J. Influence of polyphenols on bacterial biofilm formation and quorum-sensing. *Z. Naturforsch. C* **2003**, *58*, 879–884. [CrossRef] [PubMed]

35. Adonizio, A.L. *Anti-Quorum Sensing Agents from South Florida Medicinal Plants and Their Attenuation of Pseudomonas aeruginosa Pathogenicity*; Florida International University: Miami, FL, USA, 2008.

36. Shuaibu, M.N.; Pandey, K.; Wuyep, P.A.; Yanagi, T.; Hirayama, K.; Ichinose, A.; Tanaka, T.; Kouno, I. Castalagin from *Anogeissus leiocarpus* mediates the killing of *Leishmania* in vitro. *Parasitol. Res.* **2008**, *103*, 1333–1338. [CrossRef] [PubMed]

37. Chaabi, M.; Benayache, S.; Benayache, F.; N'Gom, S.; Koné, M.; Anton, R.; Weniger, B.; Lobstein, A. Triterpenes and polyphenols from *Anogeissus leiocarpus* (Combretaceae). *Biochem. Syst. Ecol.* **2007**, *36*, 59–62. [CrossRef]

38. Gloyne, L.S.; Grant, G.D.; Perkins, A.V.; Powell, K.L.; McDermott, C.M.; Johnson, P.V.; Anderson, G.J.; Kiefel, M.; Anoopkumar-Dukie, S. Pyocyanin-induced toxicity in A549 respiratory cells is causally linked to oxidative stress. *Toxicol. In Vitro* **2011**, *25*, 1353–1358. [CrossRef] [PubMed]

39. Tamura, Y.; Suzuki, S.; Kijima, M.; Takahashi, T.; Nakamura, M. Effect of proteolytic enzyme on experimental infection of mice with *Pseudomonas aeruginosa*. *J. Vet. Med. Sci.* **1992**, *54*, 597–599. [CrossRef] [PubMed]

40. Muller, M. Premature cellular senescence induced by pyocyanin, a redox-active *Pseudomonas aeruginosa* toxin. *Free Radic. Biol. Med.* **2006**, *41*, 1670–1677. [CrossRef] [PubMed]

41. Muller, M.; Li, Z.; Maitz, P.K. *Pseudomonas* pyocyanin inhibits wound repair by inducing premature cellular senescence: Role for p38 mitogen-activated protein kinase. *Burns* **2009**, *35*, 500–508. [CrossRef] [PubMed]

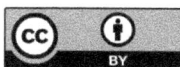

medicines

MDPI

Article

Antidermatophytic Activity of the Fruticose Lichen *Usnea orientalis*

Ashutosh Pathak [1], Dalip Kumar Upreti [2] and Anupam Dikshit [1,*]

[1]   Biological Product Lab, Department of Botany, University of Allahabad, Allahabad 211002, India;
      ashupathaks@rediffmail.com
[2]   Lichenology Laboratory, CSIR-National Botanical Research Institute, Rana Pratap Marg, Lucknow 226001,
      India; upretidknbri@gmail.com
*   Correspondence: anupambplau@rediffmail.com; Tel.: +91-532-2546200; Fax: +91-532-2461887

Academic Editor: James D. Adams
Received: 2 May 2016; Accepted: 1 September 2016; Published: 12 September 2016

Abstract: In the present study, the new biological sources in the form of lichen *Usnea orientalis* Motyka was screened for its antidermatophytic potential. Six species of dermatophytes were chosen on the basis of their prevalence for antidermatophytic assays, and the Clinical Laboratory Standard Institute (CLSI)-recommended broth microdilution procedure was used to detect the efficacy of extract against dermatophytes. Thin layer chromatography of lichen extracts reveals the presence of two secondary metabolites viz. salazinic acid and usnic acid. *U. orientalis* extract exhibited promising antidermatophytic activity against all tested pathogens. Amongst all tested pathogens, *Epidermophyton floccosum* exhibited most susceptibility towards extract, whereas *Trichophyton mentagrophytes* exhibited the least susceptibility. Topical application of *U. orientalis* extract might be helpful in the cure of dermal infections.

Keywords: antidermatophytic; dermatophytes; DPPH; Lichen

1. Introduction

Lichen thallus (a composite organism) is mainly composed of mycobiont and photobiont in a mutualistic relationship [1]. Lichens are known for their secondary metabolites, which are quite unique to them and have several properties such as photoprotection, allelopathy, and antioxidant, antimicrobial, and antiviral activities [2]. The genus *Usnea* is well known for the worldwide distribution and for the role of secondary metabolite, i.e., usnic acid, in medicines. More than 300 species of genus *Usnea* were reported throughout the world, of which 57 are from India [3]. *Usnea orientalis* Motyka (fruticose and corticolous lichen) was used ethno-medicinally in urinary tract problems, swelling, and edema [4]. Cutaneous infections caused by fungi generally produce boggy nodular swelling called kerion [5]. Cutaneous mycoses (skin infection) caused by filamentous keratinophilic fungi known as dermatophytes, composed of the three genera *Trichophyton*, *Microsporum*, and *Epidermophyton* [6]. In humans, about 30 species of dermatophytes have been identified as pathogens [7]. Dermatophytes are cosmopolitan in distribution. Several reports from different parts of the world have reported the occurrence of dermatophytes. A study involving 16 European countries showed that 35%–40% of the analyzed individuals had infection of the foot (tinea pedis) caused by dermatophytes [8]. A study in the US revealed that between 22% and 55% had hair scalp infection of dermatophytes [9]. Another study conducted in Brazil showed that *Trichophyton rubrum*, *Microsporum canis*, and *Epidermophyton floccosum* were the most prevalent species infecting humans in developing countries [10]. The World Health Organization estimated that dermatophytes affect about 25% of the world population [6]. Apart from wide prevalence, the dermatophytes have exhibited resistance against griseofulvin, terbinafine, and fluconazole [6,11–14]. Although the prevalence of drug resistance in dermatophytes is rare, recurrence in patients is common with 60%–80% [5]. Based on the aforementioned literature, the new biological source in the form of *U. orientalis* was screened for its antidermatophytic property.

2. Material and Methods

2.1. Preparation and Percent Yield of Extract

Lichen thalli were collected from Koti, Chakrata district, Uttarakhand, India and identified with the help of relevant keys [15]. The voucher specimen was deposited in the Botanical Survey of India, Allahabad, India: *U. orientalis* (Accession No. BSA-8760). Two grams of air-dried thallus (vegetative as well as fruiting) was washed thoroughly using tap water followed by distilled water and pat-dried. Then, thalli were subjected to cold extraction of secondary metabolites in 50 mL of acetone. Subsequently, the solvent was filtered by Whatman No. 1 filter paper after 48 h.

The weight of crude extract obtained was 0.16 g after vacuum drying the filtrate via rotary evaporator. Percent yield of crude extract was calculated according to the equation below:

$$\text{Percent yield (\%)} = (\text{Dry weight of extract}/\text{Dry weight of sample}) \times 100.$$

Stock solution (50 mg/mL) of crude extract was prepared in dimethyl sulphoxide (DMSO) for the evaluation of antidermatophytic and free radical scavenging activity.

2.2. Thin Layer Chromatography of Extract

Solvent A (Toluene (180 mL) 1,4 dioxane (45 mL): Acetic acid (5 mL)) and Solvent C (Toluene (170 mL): Acetic acid (30 mL)) was used as mobile phase, whereas silica-coated aluminum plate (TLC Silica gel 60 F254, Merck KGaA, Darmstadt, Germany) was used as stationary phase and Usnic acid (Chemical Industry Co., Ltd., Tokyo, Japan) was taken as standard [16].

2.3. Test Pathogens and Inocula Preparation

Fungal cultures of *Epidermophyton floccosum* (MTCC No. 7880), *Microsporum canis* (MTCC No. 3270), *M. fulvum* (MTCC No. 7684), *M. gypseum* (MTCC No. 2867), *Trichophyton rubrum* (MTCC No. 296), and *T. mentagrophytes* (MTCC No. 7687) were procured from Microbial Type Culture Collection and Gene Bank (MTCC), Chandigarh, India, and were subcultured on Sabouraud Dextrose Agar (SDA) medium under laminar flow cabinet (Laminar flow ultra clean air unit, Micro-Filt, Pune, India). Inocula were prepared in saline media and then adjusted to a 0.5 McFarland standard, corresponding to ca 0.5×10^6 CFU/mL, and transmittance of inocula prepared were 70%–72% at 520 nm for each pathogen [17].

2.4. Antifungal Assay for Opportunistic Filamentous Fungi

2.4.1. Determination of Fungistatic Concentration

Antifungal susceptibility test was performed according to the Clinical Laboratory Standard Institute (CLSI)-recommended broth microdilution method in RPMI-1640 medium HEPES modification (Sigma Aldrich, St. Louis, MO, USA) supplemented with MOPS buffer (3-morphollinopropane-1-sulfonic acid) (Qualigens Fine Chemicals, Mumbai, India) [18]. Brief steps involved per plate were as follows: Inocula prepared was diluted 1:50 times in testing media, i.e., RPMI 1640; the test was performed in 96-well flat bottom microtiter plates; Column 1 was named as negative control consisting of 100 µL of RPMI-1640 broth media and 100 µL of inocula prepared in formaldehyde (less than 0.5%); Column 2 was named as broth control consisting of 200 µL of media; Columns 3 and 4, 6 and 7, and 9 and 10 were vertically diluted with extract having a final concentration of 1.25 to 0.009 mg/mL and named as treated; Column 5, 8, and 11 were taken as positive controls and contained only 100 µL of inocula and 100 µL of RPMI-1640 broth media, respectively; Column 12 was named as extract control and contained vertically diluted extract in the aforementioned concentrations. To nullify the effect of extract color, optical density (O.D.) of the extract control was subtracted from treated columns corresponding to extract treated [19]. Percent inhibition was calculated using following equation:

$$\text{Per cent Inhibition (\%)} = ((\text{O.D. positive control} - \text{O.D. extract-treated}) / (\text{O.D. positive control})) \times 100.$$

Minimum inhibition concentrations (MICs) was calculated based on optical density recorded with a spectrophotometer (SpectraMax Plus[384], Molecular Devices Corporation, Orleans Drive, Sunnyvale, CA, USA) at 530 nm after 96 h of incubation at $30 \pm 2\,^{\circ}\text{C}$ (Figure 1).

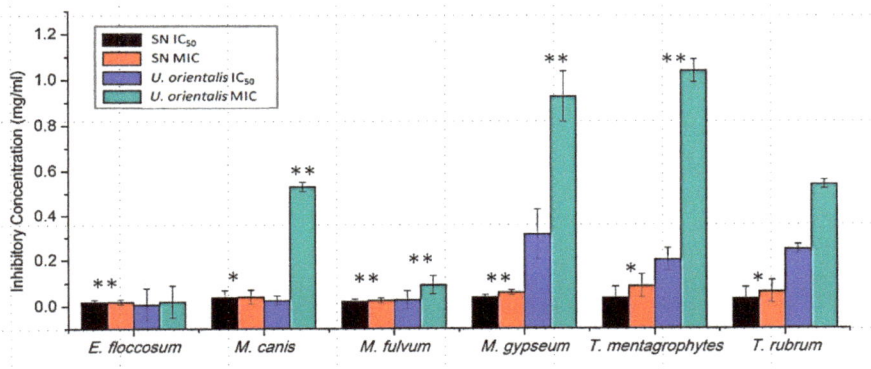

Figure 1. Antidermatophytic activity *U. orientalis* extract compared with Sertaconazole nitrate. Error bars show the standard error mean. ** Level of significance ≤ 0.01. * Level of significance ≤ 0.05.

The antifungal activity of the chemical drug Sertaconazole nitrateBP (SN) (Glenmark Pharmaceuticals, Nasik, India) was taken as the reference standard. An amount of 50 mg/mL of stock solution of SN was prepared and tested at the same concentrations as the *U. orientalis* extract.

2.4.2. Determination of Fungicidal Concentration

A portion of 20 µL of *U. orientalis*-treated columns from the above MIC wells were transferred into 7-mL tubes of a fresh RPMI 1640 medium. Tubes were incubated at $30 \pm 2\,^{\circ}\text{C}$ for 4 weeks and checked for the turbidity. The aforementioned procedure was performed with SN, and the concentration at which no turbidity has been achieved was defined as the minimum fungicidal concentration (MFC) [20,21].

2.5. Statistical Analysis

An independent sample *t*-test was performed between the positive control and sertacoazole-treated dermatophytes; and between the positive control and extract-treated dermatophytes for the measure of Levene's test for equality of variances and *t*-test for equality of means via SPSS v20.

3. Results and Discussion

3.1. Percent Yield of Extract

Percent yield of extract obtained from *U. orientalis* thallus was 8%.

3.2. Thin Layer Chromatography

A light yellow turning into a green-colored spot was observed and confirmed as usnic acid in *U. orientalis* extract and the other compound was salazinic acid. The chromatographic study confirmed the presence of two compounds viz. usnic acid and salazinic acid in the *U. orientalis* extract.

3.3. Antifungal Test for Opportunistic Filamentous Fungi

U. orientalis, fruticose lichen, contains usnic and salazinic acid and is used ethno-medicinally in swelling. The *U. orientalis* extract was tested for its efficacy against six dermatophytic species and compared with sertaconazole nitrate. Sertaconazole nitrate is a highly active chemical drug having low fungistatic and fungicidal activities, but it causes inflammation and itching in patients [22]. Due to the side effects of SN and the development of resistance in dermatophytes against first-line clinical drugs, there is a need for new antidermatophytic compounds. The antidermatophytic activity of SN and *U. orientalis* were represented graphically in the form of IC_{50} (50% inhibitory concentration) and MIC (minimum inhibitory concentration) values were represented graphically in Figure 1.

E. floccosum exhibited equal susceptibility towards SN and *U. orientalis* extract with an MIC value equivalent to 0.021 mg/mL and an MFC value equivalent to 0.039 mg/mL. The IC_{50} value for *E. floccosum* was achieved at 0.009 mg/mL against *U. orientalis* and 0.020 mg/mL against SN. *M. gypseum* was found least susceptible among *Microsporum* spp. with IC_{50} = 0.040 mg/mL; MIC = 0.062 mg/mL; MFC = 0.078 mg/mL against SN and IC_{50} = 0.316 mg/mL; MIC = 0.927 mg/mL; MFC = 1.250 mg/mL against *U. orientalis*. *M. fulvum* was found most susceptible among *Microsporum* spp. with IC_{50} = 0.022 mg/mL; MIC = 0.027 mg/mL; MFC = 0.039 mg/mL against SN and IC_{50} = 0.029 mg/mL; MIC = 0.094 mg/mL; MFC = 0.156 mg/mL against *U. orientalis*. The IC_{50}, MIC, and MFC for *M. canis* were obtained at 0.040 mg/mL, 0.043 mg/mL, and 0.078 mg/mL for SN and 0.027 mg/mL, 0.531 mg/mL, and 0.625 mg/mL for *U. orientalis* extract.

The IC_{50}, MIC, and MFC for *T. rubrum* were achieved at 0.033 mg/mL, 0.064 mg/mL, and 0.078 mg/mL against SN and 0.249 mg/mL, 0.54 mg/mL, and 0.625 mg/mL against *U. orientalis* extract. *T. mentagrophytes* was found least susceptible amongst all tested pathogens with IC_{50} = 0.037 mg/mL, MIC = 0.09 mg/mL, and MFC = 0.156 mg/mL against SN and IC_{50} = 0.204 mg/mL, MIC = 1.04 mg/mL, and MFC = 1.25 mg/mL against *U. orientalis* extract. The efficacy of *U. orientalis* extract is equivalent to sertaconazole nitrate against *E. floccosum*, but was found to be less effective against all other dermatophytes.

In another study, extracts of *U. florida* exhibited an MIC between 0.050 and 0.100 mg/mL against *M. gypseum*, *T. mentagrophytes*, and *T. rubrum* [23]. In the present study *U. orientalis* exhibited a MIC between 0.531 and 1.04 mg/mL and was found to be less active than *U. florida*. The ethno-medicinal use of *U. orientalis* extract in swelling caused by dermatophyte infection might be cured, but in vivo efficacy and potency of the lichen extract needs to be investigated.

3.4. Statistical Analysis

The level of significance was calculated in terms of *p*-value. Results obtained were statistically significant except between *U. orientalis* treatments and control *T. rubrum* (*p*-value = 0.19) and *U. orientalis* treatments and control *E. floccosum* (*p*-value = 0.19); *p*-values calculated for SN-treated *E. floccosum*, *M. fulvum*, and *M. gypseum* were less than 0.01, whereas, for *M. canis*, *T. mentagrophytes*, and *T. rubrum*, *p*-values were less than 0.05. *p*-value calculated for *U. orientalis* treated all pathogens except *T. rubrum*, *which* showed a level of significance less than 0.01 (Figure 1).

4. Conclusions

U. orientalis extract exhibited broad-range antidermatophytic activity against all three genera of dermatophytes, and usnic acid (a well-known antifungal compound) was present in the lichen extract. Topical application of lichen extract might be helpful in the cure of cutaneous infections.

Acknowledgments: Gopal Prasad Sinha, Head of Office, Central Regional Centre, Botanical Survey of India, Allahabad for accepting the voucher specimens of Lichens, and University Grant Commission (UGC) New Delhi, India, for financial assistance.

Author Contributions: Dalip Kumar Upreti identified the lichen; Ashutosh Pathak, Dalip Kumar Upreti and Anupam Dikshit designed the experiments, analyzed the results and proof reading of the manuscript; Ashutosh Pathak collected the lichen thallus, performed the experiments and wrote the manuscript.

Conflicts of Interest: The authors declare no conflict of interest.

References

1. Hawksworth, D.L. Freshwater and marine lichen-forming. In *Aquatic Mycology across the Millennium*; Hyde, K.D., Ho, W.H., Pointing, S.B., Eds.; Fungal Diversity: Hong Kong, China, 2000; Volume 5.

2. Molnar, K.; Farkas, E. Current results on Biological Activities of Lichen Secondary Metabolites: A Review. *Z. Naturforschung C* **2010**, *65*, 157–173. [CrossRef]

3. Shukla, P.; Upreti, D.K.; Tewari, L.M. Secondary metabolite variability in genus *Usnea* in India: A potential source for bioprospection. *J. Environ. Sci. Technol.* **2015**, *2*, 44–55.

4. Wang, L.S.; Qian, Z.G. *Pictorial Handbook to Medicinal Lichens in Chin*; Yunnan Provincial Science and Technology Publishers: Kunming, China, 2013.

5. Dias, M.F.R.G.; Quaresma-Santos, M.V.P.; Bernardes-Filho, F.; Amorim, A.G.F.; Schechtman, R.C.; Azulay, D.R. Update on therapy for superficial mycoses: Review article part 1. *An. Bras. Dermatol.* **2013**, *88*, 764–774. [CrossRef] [PubMed]

6. Peres, N.T.A.; Maranhão, F.C.A.; Rossi, A.; Martinez-Rossi, N.M. Dermatophytes: Host-pathogen interaction and antifungal resistance. *An. Bras. Dermatol.* **2010**, *85*, 657–667. [CrossRef] [PubMed]

7. White, T.C.; Oliver, B.G.; Graser, Y.; Henn, M.R. Generating and testing molecular hypotheses in the dermatophytes. *Eukaryot. Cell* **2008**, *7*, 1238–1245. [CrossRef] [PubMed]

8. Burzykowski, T.; Molenberghs, G.; Abeck, D.; Haneke, E.; Hay, R.; Katsambas, A.; Roseeuw, D.; van de Kerkhof, P.; van Aelst, R.; Marynissen, G. High prevalence of foot diseases in Europe: Results of the Achilles Project. *Mycoses* **2003**, *46*, 496–505. [CrossRef] [PubMed]

9. Abdel-Rahman, S.M.; Simon, S.; Wright, K.J.; Ndjountche, L.; Gaedigk, A. Tracking *Trichophyton tonsurans* through a large urban child care center: Defining infection prevalence and transmission patterns by molecular strain typing. *Pediatrics* **2006**, *118*, 2365–2373. [CrossRef] [PubMed]

10. Heidrich, D.; Garcia, M.R.; Stopiglia, C.D.O.; Magagnin, C.M.; Daboit, T.C.; Vetoratto, G.; Schwartz, J.; Amaro, T.G.; Scroferneker, M.L. Dermatophytosis: A 16-year retrospective study in a metropolitan area in southern Brazil. *J. Infect. Dev. Ctries.* **2015**, *9*, 865–871. [CrossRef] [PubMed]

11. Stephenson, J. Investigators seeking new ways to stem rising tide of resistant fungi. *J. Am. Med. Assoc.* **1997**, *277*, 5–6. [CrossRef]

12. Wingfield, A.B.; Fernandez-Obregon, A.C.; Wignall, F.S.; Greer, D.L. Treatment of tinea imbricata: A randomized clinical trial using griseofulvin, terbinafine, itraconazole and fluconazole. *Br. J. Dermatol.* **2004**, *150*, 119–126. [CrossRef] [PubMed]

13. Smith, K.J.; Warnock, D.W.; Kennedy, C.T.; Johnson, E.M.; Hopwood, V.; van Cutsem, J.; Vanden Bossche, H. Azole resistance in *Candida albicans*. *Med. Mycol.* **1986**, *24*, 133–144. [CrossRef]

14. Orozco, A.; Higginbotham, L.; Hitchcock, C.; Parkinson, T.; Falconer, D.; Ibrahim, A.; Ghannoum, M.A.; Filler, S.G. Mechanism of fluconazole resistance in *Candida krusei*. *Antimicrob. Agents Chemother.* **1998**, *42*, 2645–2649. [PubMed]

15. Awasthi, D.D. *A compendium of the Macrolichens from India, Nepal and Sri Lanka*; Bishen Singh Mahendra Pal Singh: Dehradun, India, 2007.

16. Orange, A.; James, P.W.; White, F.J. *Microchemical Methods for Identification of Lichens*; British Lichen Society: London, UK, 2001.

17. Santos, D.A.; Barros, M.E.S.; Hamdan, J.S. Establishing a method of inoculum preparation for susceptibility testing of *Trichophyton rubrum* and *Trichophyton mentagrophytes*. *J. Clin. Microbial.* **2006**, *44*, 98–101. [CrossRef] [PubMed]

18. Rex, J.H.; Alexander, B.D.; Andes, D.; Arthington-Skaggs, B.; Brown, S.D.; Chaturveli, V.; Espinel-Ingroff, A.; Ghannoum, M.A.; Knapp, C.C.; Motyl, M.R.; et al. *Reference Method for Broth Dilution Antifungal Susceptibility Testing of Filamentous Fungi, Approved Standard*, 2nd ed.; M38A2 28(16); Clinical and Laboratory Standard Institute (CLSI): Wayne, PA, USA, 2008.

19. Pathak, A.; Shukla, S.K.; Pandey, A.; Mishra, R.K.; Kumar, R.; Dikshit, A. In vitro antibacterial activity of ethno medicinally used lichens against three wound infecting genera of Enterobacteriaceae. *Proc. Natl. Acad. Sci. India Sect. B Biol. Sci.* **2015**. [CrossRef]

20. Veinovic, G.; Cerar, T.; Strle, F.; Lotric-Furlan, S.; Maraspin, V.; Cimperman, J.; Ruzic-Sabjic, E. In vitro susceptibility of European human *Borrelia burgdorferi* sensu stricto strains to antimicrobial agents. *Int. J. Antimicrob. Agents* **2013**, *41*, 288–291. [CrossRef] [PubMed]

21. Pathak, A.; Mishra, R.K.; Shukla, S.K.; Kumar, R.; Pandey, M.; Pandey, M.; Qidwai, A. In vitro evaluation of antidermatophytic activity of five lichens. *Cogent Biol.* **2016**. [CrossRef]

22. Liebel, F.; Lyte, P.; Garay, M.; Babad, J.; Southall, M.D. Anti-inflammatory and anti-itch activity of sertaconazole nitrate. *Arch. Dermatol. Res.* **2006**, *298*, 191–199. [CrossRef] [PubMed]

23. Schmeda-Hirschmann, G.; Tapia, A.; Lima, B.; Pertino, M.; Sortino, M.; Zacchino, S.; Arias, A.R.; Feresin, G.E. A new antifungal and antiprotozoal depside from the Andean lichen *Protousnea poeppigii*. *Phytother. Res.* **2008**, *22*, 349–355. [CrossRef] [PubMed]

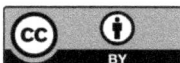

MDPI

Article

Cytotoxic and Antimicrobial Constituents from the Essential Oil of *Lippia alba* (Verbenaceae)

Nara O. dos Santos [1], Renata C. Pascon [1], Marcelo A. Vallim [1], Carlos R. Figueiredo [2], Marisi G. Soares [3], João Henrique G. Lago [1,4,*] and Patricia Sartorelli [1,*]

[1] Instituto de Ciências Ambientais, Químicas e Farmacêuticas, Universidade Federal de São Paulo, Diadema 09972-270, SP, Brazil; nara.oshiro@gmail.com (N.O.d.S.); renata.pascon@gmail.com (R.C.P.); marcelo.vallim@gmail.com (M.A.V.)

[2] Disciplina de Biologia Celular, Departamento de Micro, Imuno e Parasitologia, Universidade Federal de São Paulo, Sao Paulo 04021-001, SP, Brazil; rogernty@hotmail.com

[3] Instituto de Química, Universidade Federal de Alfenas, Alfenas 37130-000, MG, Brazil; marisigs@gmail.com

[4] Centro de Ciências Naturais e Humanas, Universidade Federal do ABC, Santo Andre 09210-180, SP, Brazil

* Correspondence: joao.lago@unifesp.br (J.H.G.L.); psartorelli@unifesp.br (P.S.); Tel.: +55-11-3385-3473 (J.H.G.L. & P.S.); Fax: +55-11-3319-3400 (J.H.G.L. & P.S.)

Academic Editor: James D. Adams

Received: 30 June 2016; Accepted: 9 August 2016; Published: 12 August 2016

Abstract: Backgroud: *Lippia alba* (Verbenaceae) is a plant widely used in folk medicine to treat various diseases. The present work deals with the chemical composition of the crude essential oil extracted from leaves of *L. alba* and evaluation of its antimicrobial and cytotoxic activities. **Methods:** Leaves of *L. alba* were extracted by hydrodistillation and analyzed by gas chromatography/mass spectrometry (GC/MS) as well as by nuclear magnetic resonance (NMR) spectroscopy. Cytotoxic and antimicrobial activities of crude essential oil were evaluated in vitro using MTT and broth microdilution assays, respectively. **Results:** Chemical analysis afforded the identification of 39 substances corresponding to 99.45% of the total oil composition. Concerning the main compounds, monoterpenes nerol/geraniol and citral correspond to approximately 50% of crude oil. The cytotoxic activity of obtained essential oil against several tumor cell lines showed IC_{50} values ranging from 45 to 64 µg/mL for B16F10Nex2 (murine melanoma) and A549 (human lung adenocarcinoma). In the antimicrobial assay, was observed that all tested yeast strains, except *C. albicans*, were sensitive to crude essential oil. MIC values were two to four-folds lower than those determined to bacterial strains. **Conclusion:** Analysis of chemical composition of essential oils from leaves of *L. alba* suggested a new chemotype nerol/geraniol and citral. Based in biological evidences, a possible application for studied oil as an antifungal in medicine, as well as in agriculture, is described.

Keywords: *Lippia alba*; essential oil; cytotoxic activity; antimicrobial activity

1. Introduction

The Verbenaceae family, with tropical and subtropical distribution, is composed of approximately 90 genera, including *Lippia* [1], with more than 200 species of herbaceous plants, small shrubs, and trees [2,3]. Most of these species have traditionally been used in the treatment of gastrointestinal and respiratory diseases [4]. Several pharmacological aspects have been ascribed to the genus *Lippia*, including antimicrobial, antifungal, antimalarial, larvicidal, antispasmodic, analgesic, anti-inflammatory, and antipyretic activities. *Lippia alba* (Mill.) N.E. Brown is native to the Americas widely distributed across the Southern United States and Northern Argentina [5]. In Brazil, this plant is popularly known as lemon balm [6,7] and have been used in folk medicine for the treatment of various diseases, such as gastric diseases, diarrhea, fever, asthma, cough, and soothing, antispasmodic, and emenagoga [2,8–13]. As other species from the same genus, phytochemicals from *L. alba* exhibited antibacterial, antifungal, antiviral, antiprotozoal, analgesic, anti-inflammatory, cytotoxic, antioxidant, and acaricidal activities [5]. Essential oils obtained from the leaves of *L. alba* were previously studied and three different chemotypes were reported: myrcene/citral, limonene/citral and limonene/carvone [14]. Zoghbi et al. [15] classified three other chemotypes: eucalyptol/limonene, limonene/carvone, and citral/germacrene-D. In addition to these volatile compounds, other monoterpenes and phenylpropanoids have been described as main metabolites in the essential oils from *L. alba*: linalool, β-caryophyllene, tagetone, myrcene, γ-terpinene, camphor, estragole, eucalyptol, camphor, limonene, and piperitone [12–18]. This variability has been explained due to factors such as seasons, flowering time, plant age, amount of precipitation, geographic and climatic factors [8,12,19], as well as the part of the studied plant, extraction method, soil characteristics, and the genetic variability of these plants [12,20–23]. These differences may lead to a different oil composition and, therefore, to different pharmacological effects [9,12]. As part of our continuous study with volatile oils from Brazilian species [24–26], the present work deals with the chemical composition of the essential oil from leaves of the Brazilian species of *L. alba*, as well as the cytotoxic and antimicrobial evaluation of crude essential oil.

2. Materials and Methods

2.1. General Experimental Procedures

^{1}H and ^{13}C NMR spectra of crude oil were registered, respectively, at 300 and 75 MHz into a Ultrashield 300 Advance III spectrometer (Bruker, Fremont, CA, USA) using CDCl$_3$ (Aldrich, St. Louis, MO, USA) as solvent and tetramethylsilane (TMS) as internal standard. Gas chromatograms were obtained on a GC-2010 gas chromatograph (Shimadzu, Kyoto, Japan) equipped with an FID-detector and AOC-20i automatic injector (Shimadzu, Kyoto, Japan) using a RtX-5 (5% phenyl, 95% polydimethylsiloxane-30 m × 0.32 mm × 0.25 μm film thickness, Restek (Bellefonte, PA, USA)) capillary column. These analyses were performed by injecting 1.0 μL of a 1.0 mg/mL solution of volatile oil in CH$_2$Cl$_2$ in a split mode (1:10) employing helium as the carrier gas (1 mL/min) under the following conditions: injector and detector temperatures of 220 °C and 250 °C, respectively; oven programmed temperature from 40 to 240 °C at 3 °C/min, holding 5 min at 240 °C. The percentage compositions of the oil samples were computed by internal normalization from the flame ionization detector gas chromatography (GC-FID) peak areas without using correction for response factors. Gas chromatography coupled to low resolution electronic impact mass spectrometry (GC-LREIMS) analysis was conducted in a GC-17A chromatograph interfaced with a MS-QP-5050A mass spectrometer (Shimadzu, Kyoto, Japan). The LREIMS operating conditions were an ionization voltage of 70 eV and an ion source temperature of 230 °C with the same conditions described above. The identification of the individual compounds was performed by comparison of retention indexes (determined relatively to the retention times of a series of *n*-alkanes) and comparison of recorded mass spectra with those available in the system [27].

2.2. Plant Material

Leaves of *L. alba* were collected at Instituto Plantarum de Estudos da Flora in Nova Odessa city (coordinates 22°46′46″ S e 47°18′49″ O), São Paulo State, Brazil in 2014. Botanical identification was performed by Dr. Harri Lorenzi. The voucher of the studied species has been deposited in the Herbarium Plantarum (HPL) at number Lorenzi 1.713.

2.3. Essential Oil Extraction and Analysis

Fresh leaves (150 g) of *L. alba* were submitted to a steam distillation in a Clevenger-type apparatus over 5 h to afford 931 mg of the crude essential oil. The obtained oil was immediately analyzed by GC-FID and GC-LREIMS.

2.4. Cell Lines

The murine melanoma cell line B16F10 was originally obtained from the Ludwig Institute for Cancer Research (São Paulo, Brazil). The melanotic B16F10Nex2 subline, characterized at the Experimental Oncology Unit (UNIFESP-Federal University of São Paulo), is characterized by low immunogenicity and moderate virulence. Human breast cancer cell line (MCF-7), human lung adenocarcinoma (A549), and human umbilical vein endothelial (HUVEC) were obtained from the Ludwig Institute for Cancer Research.

2.5. In Vitro Cytotoxic Activity

The essential oil extracted from leaves of *L. alba* was dissolved in dimethyl sulfoxide (DMSO) to the final concentration of 10 mg/mL, diluted in RPMI medium containing 10% fetal calf serum ranging from 100 to 0 µg/mL and incubated with 1×10^4 cells in a 96-well plate. After 18 h of incubation, cell viability was measured using the Cell Proliferation Kit I (MTT) (Sigma, St. Louis, MI, USA), an MTT-based colorimetric assay [27,28]. Readings were made with a plate reader at 570 nm. All experiments were performed in triplicate.

2.6. Media, Antibiotics, and Growth Conditions

Yeast were cultivated on agar plates containing YPD (1% yeast extract, 2% peptone, 2% dextrose, and 2% agar) or RPMI1640 (Sigma). Gram-negative bacteria were grown in LB (0.5% yeast extract, 1% tryptone, 1% NaCl, and 2% agar) and Gram-positive bacteria were tested in BHI (Himedia, Mumbai, India). Fluconazole (Sigma) was used as the positive control for yeast and chloramphenicol (Sigma) was the positive control for bacteria. Crude essential oil from *L. alba* was diluted in DMSO or saline (0.9%) plus Tween 80 (0.5%) and spotted on 5 mm sterile filter paper [25].

2.7. Microorganisms Strains

The bacteria and yeast species used in this work are described in the Table 1.

Table 1. Target strains used for antimicrobial activity assays.

Species	Designation
Yeast	
Candida dubliniensis	ATCC 7978
Candida tropicalis	ATCC 13803
Candida glabrata	ATCC 90030
Candida parapsilosis	Clinical isolate 68
Candida krusei	Clinical isolate 9602
Candida albicans	CBMAI * 560
Cryptococcus grubii (A)	ATCC 208821
Cryptococcus gattii (B)	ATCC MYA-4563
Cryptococcus gattii (C)	ATCC MYA-4560
Cryptococcus neoformans (D)	ATCC MYA-4567
Saccharomyces cerevisiae	ATCC 201389
Bacteria	
Escherichia coli	-
Serratia marcescens	CBMAI * 469
Pseudomonas aeruginosa	CBMAI * 602
Staphylococcus epidermidis	CBMAI * 604
Enterococcus faecalis	-

* CBMAI: Coleção Brasileira de Microrganismos do Ambiente e Indústria.

2.8. Disk Diffusion Assay

Antimicrobial activity of essential oil from leaves of *L. alba* was evaluated using the disk diffusion method according to the Clinical and Laboratory Standards Institute (CLSI, OPAS M2-A8) with modifications. Thin agar plates were prepared with 10 mL of YPD (yeast), LB (Gram-negative) and BHI (Gram-positive) media. Three milliliters of liquid cultures were grown at 30 °C with aeration

(150 rpm) overnight on YPD (yeast), LB (Gram-negative), or BHI (Gram-positive). A top agar was prepared by mixing 100 μL of each culture with 10 mL of soft agar medium for confluent plates (YPD, LB or BHI plus 1% agar) and poured on top of the thin agar (2% agar medium). Sterilized 5 mm filter paper disks were then impregnated with 20 μL of crude essential oil diluted in DMSO. The disks were placed on top of agar plates and incubated at 30 °C for 24 or 48 h depending on the microorganism. Fluconazole (1 mg) and chloramphenicol (200 μg) were used as positive controls for yeast and bacteria, respectively. Negative control was prepared by impregnating the paper disks with the same amount of DMSO used to dilute the essential oil. All tests were performed in triplicate. Tested strains were selected since they represent clinical important microbes and were previously tested in other studies conducted by our research group [25].

2.9. Minimum Inhibitory Concentration

Microdilution tests were conducted according to the Clinical and Laboratory Standards Institute (CLSI), OPAS1 M27-A2 for yeasts and OPAS M7-A6 for bacteria according to literature [25] with slight modifications. Briefly, minimum inhibitory concentration (MIC) values were determined using microtiter plates (96 wells) with a total volume of 100 μL. Microorganisms were cultured in test tubes filled with 3 mL medium RPMI 1640 (Sigma, St. Louis, MI, USA) for yeast and BHI (Sigma, St. Louis, MI, USA) for bacteria, overnight at 30 °C in a rotary shaker (150 rpm). The cultures were diluted and adjusted to 1–2×10^2 CFU/mL, which was confirmed by viability counts on YPD and BHI plates (100 μL of diluted cells). Crude essential oil and reference standards were serial diluted (two-fold) and added to each well. A sterilization control containing medium only and growth control containing cell, DMSO (10 μL), or saline (10 μL), and Tween 80 were included as negative and positive controls, respectively. Depending on the microorganism the microtiter plates were then incubated at 30 °C for 24 or 48 h. Microorganism growth was determined by reading the absorbance at 530 nm in a plate reader Logen MT-960 (Tecan, Männedorf, Switzerland) and the minimum inhibitory concentration was considered the lowest concentration at which at least 80% of growth was inhibited. All tests were performed in triplicate.

3. Results and Discussion

3.1. Chemical Composition of Essential Oil from L. alba

The yield of the essential oil extracted from *L. alba* was 0.21% based on the weight of the fresh leaves used in the distillation procedure. Analysis of the crude oil by gas chromatography with flame ionization detector (GC-FID) and by gas chromatography coupled to low resolution electronic impact mass spectrometry (GC-LREIMS), followed by calculation of Kovats indices, and comparison with the literature data [27] allowed the identification of 39 compounds corresponding to 99.45% (Table 2) of the crude essential oil.

Among the identified compounds, approximately 67% corresponds to monoterpenes and 19% to sesquiterpenes. The main characterized components were the isomeric monoterpenes nerol/geraniol (27.09%) and citral (21.87%), as well as 6-methyl-5-hepten-2-one (11.98%) and *E*-caryophyllene (9.25%), as showed in Figure 1. These compounds were previously found as minor metabolites in the essential oil from leaves of *L. alba* [29], suggesting the new chemotype nerol/geraniol and citral to the studied oil.

To confirm the identification of these main monoterpenes, the ^{13}C NMR spectrum of crude oil was recorded and exhibited peaks assigned to carbonyl groups of aldehydes (C-1) at δ 191.5 and 190.9 of geranial and neral, respectively. The peaks at δ 127.4/128.6 and δ 122.5/122.2 were assigned to double bonds (C-2 and C-6), whereas those at δ 164.2/164.2 and δ 132.9/133.7 were attributed to C-3 and C-7 of geranial and neral, respectively. The secondary carbons C-4 and C-5 were represented by signals δ 40.6/25.7 and 32.6/27.0. The signals of carbons C-8 (δ 17.7) and C-9 (δ 25.6) displayed the same chemical shift for neral and geranial, but the peaks observed to C-10 were observed at δ 25.1 to neral and δ 17.6 to geranial, according to literature data [30,31]. Finally, analysis of ^{1}H NMR spectrum indicated a ratio of 5:3 of geranial:neral based in the integration of the doublets at δ 9.99 (*J* = 9.0 Hz) and 9.89 (*J* = 9.0 Hz), assigned to aldehyde hydrogens (H-1).

Table 2. Chemical composition of the essential oil obtained from leaves of *L. alba*.

Compound	IK	Relative Amount
α-pinene	939	0.15
Sabinene	976	0.41
6-methy-5-hepten-2-one	985	11.98
α-phelandrene	1005	3.25
α-terpinene	1018	0.23
β-phelandrene	1031	1.67
Z-β-ocimene	1040	0.18
E-β-ocimene	1050	2.70
γ-terpinene	1062	0.03
cis-sabinene hydrate	1068	0.04
Terpinolene	1088	0.02
Linalol	1098	2.14
cis-oxide rose	1111	0.80
Dihydrolinalol	1134	0.14
Citronelal	1153	0.45
Borneol	1165	0.33
α-terpineol	1189	1.15
Citronelol	1228	4.43
nerol/geraniol	1252	27.09
citral (neral/geranial)	1267	21.87
geranyl formate	1300	1.48
Longicyclene	1373	0.11
Longifolene	1402	1.65
α-cedrene	1409	0.62
E-caryophyllene	1418	9.25
cis-thujopsene	1429	0.12
α-humulene	1454	0.82
allo-aromadendrene	1461	0.25
α-acoradiene	1463	0.04
Chamigrene	1475	0.04
germacrene-D	1480	1.67
Ar-curcumene	1483	0.38
α-zingiberene	1495	0.97
germacrene-A	1503	0.98
β-bisabolene	1509	0.20
Z-γ-bisabolene	1515	0.18
epi-longipinanol	1561	0.03
Longipinanol	1566	1.53
(6R,7R)-bisabolone	1737	0.07
Monoterpenes		67.08
Sesquiterpenes		18.91
Other compounds		13.46
Total		99.45

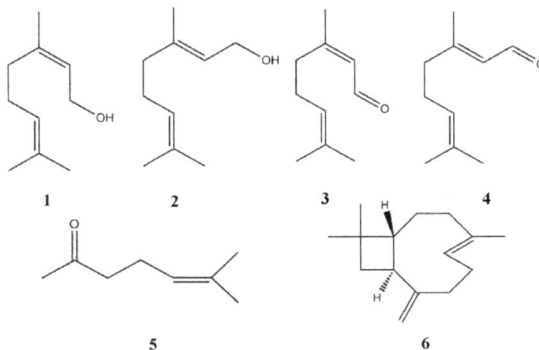

Figure 1. Structures of main compounds identified in essential oil from *L. alba*: nerol (**1**), geraniol (**2**), neral (**3**), geranial (**4**), 6-methy-5-hepten-2-one, (**5**) and *E*-caryophyllene (**6**).

3.2. Cytotoxic Activity

The essential oil from leaves of *L. alba* was evaluated for its cytotoxic activity in vitro against the lines B16F10Nex2 and A549 with IC_{50} of 45.8 µg/mL and 63.9 µg/mL, respectively, and IC_{50} higher than 100 µg/mL to the MCF-7 cell line. Comparatively, positive control cisplatin displayed IC_{50} of 52.8 µg/mL (B16F10Nex2), whereas paclitaxel showed IC_{50} of 84.3 µg/mL (A549) and 171.5 µg/mL (MCF), as showed in Table 3. Based in the obtained results, the essential oil from *L. alba* could be considered as a source of antitumor compounds, since it showed lower IC_{50} values in comparison to standard drugs in the tested cells. Additionally, the essential oil from *L. alba* was non-toxic to non-tumorigenic in HUVEC, in opposition to the cisplatin positive control, which displayed an IC_{50} value of 42.6 µg/mL.

Table 3. IC_{50} (µg/mL) values to the essential oil from leaves of *L. alba* and to positive control (cisplatin and paclitaxel) against cell lines.

Cell Line	IC_{50} (µg/mL)		
	Essential Oil	Cisplatin	Paclitaxel
B16F10Nex2	45.82 ± 4.16	52.8 ± 4.50	-
A549	63.98 ± 6.76	-	84.3 ± 6.83
MCF-7	>100	-	171.5 ± 16.39
HUVEC	>100	42.6 ± 2.25	-

In a previous study concerning the cytotoxic activity of essential oils from *L. alba* against cell lines CT26WT (murine colon carcinoma), A549 (human lung adenocarcinoma), MDA-MB-231 (human breast adenocarcinoma), CACO 2 (human colon carcinoma), and CHO (normal hamster ovary cells) no activity was observed to chemotype geraniol, whereas chemotype carvone inhibited A549 cells with IC_{50} of 47.80 µg/mL [32,33]. Otherwise, citral and carvone chemotypes of *L. alba* displayed dose-dependent cytotoxicity effect against HeLa (human cervical carcinoma) cells [34]. Regarding the major component citral, this compound exhibited antitumor activity. The effect of citral combined with retinoic acid showed inhibition of proliferation of A549 (lung carcinoma epithelial) in a dose dependent manner [35]. Additionally, antitumor properties was detected to micelle formulation of citral [36], whereas cytotoxicity against colon adenocarcinoma (HCT) and lung adenocarcinoma was described for citral, administered as a mixture of monoterpenes neral + geranial and in a combination with lysine [37]. Geraniol, another main compound found in the studied essential oil from *L. alba*, was described as an inhibitor of prostate cancer growth by targeting cell cycle and apoptosis pathways [38].

3.3. Antimicrobial Activity

Initially, disk diffusion assays were conducted with the yeasts and bacterial strains listed in Table 1 in order to screen for antimicrobial activity. Four bacterial strains (two Gram-negative and two Gram-positive) were sensitive to the essential oil from *L. alba*. In sequence, the species listed in Table 4 were tested to determine the MICs. The results showed that yeasts are considerably more sensitive to essential oil from *L. alba* than bacterial strains. At 4 mg/mL only *E. coli* showed a growth inhibition over 80%; all other strains showed an MIC of 4.0 mg/mL with growth inhibitions below 70%. Conversely, all yeast strains tested were sensitive to the essential oil from *L. alba* and the MICs calculated for them was two- to four-fold lower than those found for bacterial strains. *C. dubliniensis* was the microbial strain most sensitive to essential oil from *L. alba* (0.5 mg/mL). All yeast strains tested showed, at least, 90% of growth inhibition.

Table 4. Minimum inhibitory concentrations (MIC) for essential oil from *L. alba*. Concentrations are given in mg/mL. Numbers in parentheses denote the percentage of growth inhibition and its standard deviation.

Species	Essential Oil	Positive Control
E. coli	4.0 (98% ± 1%)	0.01 [a]
S. marcescens	4.0 (42% ± 3%)	0.01 [a]
E. faecalis	4.0 (64% ± 2%)	0.02 [a]
S. epidermidis	4.0 (56% ± 2%)	0.04 [a]
C. albicans	2.0 (99% ± 2%)	0.025 [b]
C. dubliniensis	0.5 (93% ± 2%)	0.006 [b]
C. tropicalis	2.0 (99% ± 1%)	0.05 [b]
C. glabrata	2.0 (99% ± 1%)	0.05 [b]
C. parapsilosis	2.0 (99% ± 1%)	0.006 [b]
C. krusei	2.0 (99% ± 1%)	0.05 [b]
C. grubii (A)	1.0 (99% ± 2%)	0.013 [b]
C. gattii (B)	2.0 (97% ± 2%)	0.025 [b]
C. gattii (C)	2.0 (98% ± 1%)	0.006 [b]
C. neoformans (D)	1.0 (98% ± 2%)	0.006 [b]
S. cerevisiae	2.0 (99% ± 1%)	0.013 [b]

[a] chloramphenicol; [b] fluconazole.

There are many reports in the literature about the antimicrobial effects of essential oils from *L. alba*. In our investigation the activity of this oil on bacterial growth was modest, suggesting that the tested crude oil does not play an important role as an antibacterial. However, future studies with purified fractions from this oil could uncover more significant biological activities against bacteria, as shown before by Klein et al. [39]. Essential oils from *L. alba* have been extensively reported as antifungal, especially against phyto [40–43] and human pathogens [43]. In summary, these results hold a promise of possible applications for *L. alba* essential oil as an antifungal in medicine, as well as in agriculture.

Acknowledgments: The authors wish to thank MSc. Harri Lorenzi for the collection of *Lippia alba*. Also the authors would like to thank Fundação de Amparo a Pesquisa do Estado de São Paulo-FAPESP (Project 2015/11936-2) and Conselho Nacional de Desenvolvimento Científico e Tecnológico-CNPq for providing financial support to this study. Nara O. dos Santos obtained a fellowship from Coordenação de Aperfeiçoamento de Pessoal de Nível Superior-CAPES. Patricia Sartorelli and João Henrique G. Lago received a scientific research award from CNPq.

Author Contributions: N.O.d.S., R.C.P., M.A.V., C.R.F., M.G.S. performed the experiments, contributed reagents/materials/analysis tools and wrote the manuscript. J.H.G.L. and P.S. conceived, designed the project, analyze the results and wrote the paper.

Conflicts of Interest: The authors declare that there are no conflicts of interest.

References

1. Trease, G.E.; Evans, W.C. *Pharmacognosy*, 12th ed.; Bailliere & Tindall: London, UK, 1983.

2. Pascual, M.E.; Slowing, K.; Carretero, E.; Mata, D.S.; Villar, A. *Lippia*: Traditional uses, chemistry and pharmacology: A review. *J. Ethnopharmacol.* **2001**, *76*, 201–214. [CrossRef]

3. Terblanché, F.C.; Kornelius, G. Essential oil constituents of the genus *Lippia* (Verbenaceae)—A literature review. *J. Essent. Oil Res.* **1996**, *8*, 471–485. [CrossRef]

4. Morton, J.F. *Atlas of medicinal plants of middle America: Bahamas to Yucatan*; Charles, C., Ed.; Thomas: Springfield, IL, USA, 1981.

5. Hennebelle, T.; Sahpaz, S.; Joseph, H.; Bailleul, F. Ethnopharmacology of *Lippia alba*. *J. Ethnopharmacol.* **2008**, *116*, 211–222. [CrossRef] [PubMed]

6. Jannuzzi, H.; Mattos, J.K.A.; Silva, D.B.; Gracindo, L.A.M.; Vieira, R.F. Avaliação agronômica e química de dezessete acessos de erva-cidreira (*Lippia alba* (Mill.) N.E. Brown)—Quimiotipo citral, cultivados no Distrito Federal. *Rev. Bras. Plantas Med.* **2011**, *13*, 258–264. (In Portuguese)

7. Matos, F.J.A. *Plantas Medicinais: Guia de seleção e emprego de plantas usadas em fitoterapia no Nordeste do Brasil*, 2nd ed.; UFC: Fortaleza, Brazil, 2000. (In Portuguese)

8.   Corrêa, C.B.V. Contribuição ao estudo de *Lippia alba* (Mill.) N.E. Br. ex Britt & Wilson—Erva-cidreira. *Rev. Bras. Farmacogn.* **1992**, *73*, 57–64. (In Portuguese)

9.   Matos, F.J.A. As ervas cidreiras do Nordeste do Brasil—Estudo de três quimiotipos de *Lippia alba* (Mill.) N.E. Brown (Verbenaceae). Parte II—Farmacoquímica. *Rev. Bras. Farm.* **1996**, *77*, 137–141. (In Portuguese)

10. Gupta, M. *270 Plantas Medicinales Iberoamericanas*, 1st ed.; Convenio Andrés Bello: Santafé de Bogotá, Colombia, 1995.

11. Morais, S.M.; Dantas, J.D.P.; Silva, A.R.A.; Magalhães, E.F. Plantas medicinais usadas pelos índios Tapebas do Ceará. *Rev. Bras. Farmacogn.* **2005**, *15*, 169–177. (In Portuguese) [CrossRef]

12. Tavares, E.S.; Julião, L.S.; Lopes, D.; Bizzo, H.R.; Lage, C.L.S.; Leitão, S.G. Análise do óleo essencial de folhas de três quimiotipos de *Lippia alba* (Mill.) N.E. Br. (Verbenaceae) cultivados em condições semelhantes. *Rev. Bras. Farmacogn.* **2005**, *15*, 1–5. (In Portuguese) [CrossRef]

13. Pinto, E.P.P.; Amorozo, M.C.M.; Furlan, A. Conhecimento popular sobre plantas medicinais em comunidades rurais de mata atlântica-Itacaré, BA, Brasil. *Acta Bot. Bras.* **2006**, *20*, 751–762. (In Portuguese) [CrossRef]

14. Matos, F.J.A.; Machado, M.I.L.; Craveiro, A.A.; Alencar, J.W. Essential oil composition of two chemotypes of *Lippia alba* grown in Northeast Brazil. *J. Essent. Oil Res.* **1996**, *8*, 695–698. [CrossRef]

15. Zoghbi, M.G.B.; Andrade, E.H.A.; Santos, A.S.; Silva, M.H.L.; Maia, J.G. Essential oils of *Lippia alba* (Mill.) N.E. Br. growing wild in the Brazilian Amazon. *Flavour Fragr. J.* **1998**, *13*, 47–48. [CrossRef]

16. Hennebelle, T.; Sahpaz, S.; Joseph, H.; Bailleul, F. Phenolics and iridoids of *Lippia alba*. *Nat. Prod. Commun.* **2006**, *1*, 727–730.

17. Dellacassa, E.; Soler, E.; Menéndez, P.; Moyna, P. Essential oils from *Lippia alba* (Mill.) N.E. Brown and *Aloysia chamaedrifolia* Cham. (Verbenaceae) from Uruguay. *Flavour Fragr. J.* **1990**, *5*, 107–108. [CrossRef]

18. Senatore, F.; Rigano, D. Essential oil of two *Lippia* spp. (Verbenaceae) growing wild in Guatemala. *Flavour Fragr. J.* **2001**, *16*, 169–171. [CrossRef]

19. Machado, T.F.; Pereira, R.C.A.; Batista, V.C.V. Seasonal variability of the antimicrobial activity of the essential oil of *Lippia alba*. *Rev. Ciênc. Agron.* **2014**, *45*, 515–519. [CrossRef]

20. Alea, J.A.P.; Luis, A.G.O.; Pérez, A.R.; Jorge, M.R.; Baluja, R. Composición y propriedades antibacterianas del aceite esencial de *Lippia alba* (Mill.) N.E. Brown. *Rev. Cuba. Farm.* **1996**, *30*, 1–8. (In Spanish)

21. Stashenko, E.E.; Jaramillo, B.E.; Martínez, J.R. Comparison of different extraction methods for the analysis of volatile secondary metabolites of *Lippia alba* (Mill.) N.E. Brown, grown in Colombia, and evaluation of its in vitro antioxidant activity. *J. Chromatogr. A* **2004**, *1025*, 93–103. [CrossRef] [PubMed]

22. Castro, D.M.; Ming, L.C.; Marques, M.O.M. Composição fitoquímica dos óleos essenciais de folhas da *Lippia alba* (Mill). N.E. Br. em diferentes épocas de colheita e partes do ramo. *Rev. Bras. Plantas Med.* **2002**, *4*, 75–79. (In Portuguese)

23. Viccini, L.F.; Silveira, R.S.; Vale, A.A.; Campos, J.M.S.; Reis, A.C.; Santos, M.O.; Campos, V.R.; Carpanez, A.G.; Grazul, R.M. Citral and linalool content has been correlated to DNA content in *Lippia alba* (Mill.) N.E. Brown (Verbenaceae). *Ind. Crop. Prod.* **2014**, *59*, 14–19.

24. Bou, D.D.; Lago, J.H.G.; Figueiredo, C.R.; Matsuo, A.L.; Guadagnin, R.C.; Soares, M.G.; Sartorelli, P. Cytotoxicity evaluation of essential oil, zingiberene and derivatives from leaves of *Casearia sylvestris* (Salicaceae). *Molecules* **2013**, *18*, 9477–9487. [CrossRef] [PubMed]

25. Santos, N.O.; Mariane, B.; Lago, J.H.G.; Sartorelli, P.; Rosa, W.; Soares, M.G.; da Silva, A.M.; Lorenzi, H.; Vallim, M.A.; Pascon, R.C. Assessing the chemical composition and antimicrobial activity of essential oils from Brazilian plants—*Eremanthus erythropappus* (Asteraceae), *Plectrantuns barbatus*, and *P. amboinicus* (Lamiaceae). *Molecules* **2015**, *20*, 8440–8452. [CrossRef] [PubMed]

26. Grecco, S.S.; Martins, E.G.; Girola, N.; de Figueiredo, C.R.; Matsuo, A.L.; Soares, M.G.; Bertoldo, B.C.; Sartorelli, P.; Lago, J.H.G. Chemical composition and in vitro cytotoxic effects of the essential oil from *Nectandra leucantha* leaves. *Pharm. Biol.* **2015**, *53*, 133–137. [CrossRef] [PubMed]

27. Adams, R.P. *Identification of Essential Oil Components by Gas Chromatography/Mass Spectrometry*, 4th ed.; Allured Publishing: Carol Stream, IL, USA, 2007.

28. Mosmann, T. Rapid colorimetric assay for cellular growth and survival: Application to proliferation and cytotoxicity assays. *J. Immunol. Meth.* **1983**, *65*, 55–63. [CrossRef]

29. Soares, L. Estudo tecnológico, fitoquímico e biológico de *Lippia alba* (Miller) N.E. Brown Ex Britt. & Wils. (falsa-melissa) Verbenaceae. Master's Thesis, Federal University of Santa Catarina, Florianópolis, Brazil, 2001. (In Portuguese)

30. Glamoclija, J.; Sokovic, M.; Tesevic, V.; Linde, G.A.; Colauto, N.B. Chemical characterization of *Lippia alba* essential oil: An alternative to control green molds. *Braz. J. Microbiol.* **2011**, *42*, 1537–1546. [PubMed]

31. Ragasa, C.Y.; Ha, H.K.; Hasika, M.; Maridable, J.B.; Gaspillo, P.D.; Rideout, J.A. Antimicrobial and Cytotoxic Terpenoids from *Cymbopogon citratus* Stapf. *Philipp. Scient. J.* **2008**, *45*, 111–122. [CrossRef]

32. Jeon, J.H.; Lee, C.H.; Lee, H.S. Food protective effect of geraniol and its congeners against stored food mites. *J. Food Prot.* **2009**, *72*, 1468–1471. [PubMed]

33. Gomide, M.S.; Lemos, F.O.; Lopes, M.T.P.; Alves, T.M.A.; Viccini, L.F.; Coelho, C.M. The effect of the essential oils from five different *Lippia* species on the viability of tumor cell lines. *Rev. Bras. Farmacogn.* **2013**, *23*, 895–902. [CrossRef]

34. Mesa-Arango, A.C.; Montiel-Ramos, J.; Zapata, B.; Durán, C.; Betancur-Galvis, L.; Stashenko, E. Citral and carvone chemotypes from the essential oils of Colombian *Lippia alba* (Mill.) N.E. Brown: Composition, cytotoxicity and antifungal activity. *Mem. Inst. Oswaldo Cruz* **2009**, *104*, 878–884. [CrossRef] [PubMed]

35. Farah, I.O.; Trimble, Q.; Ndebele, K.; Mawson, A. Retinoids and citral modulated cell viability, metabolic stability, cell cycle progression and distribution in the A549 lung carcinoma cell line. *Biomed. Sci. Instrum.* **2010**, *46*, 410–421. [PubMed]

36. Zeng, S.; Kapur, A.; Patankar, M.S.; Xiong, M.P. Formulation, Characterization, and Antitumor Properties of Trans- and Cis-Citral in the 4T 1 Breast Cancer Xenograft Mouse Model. *Pharm. Res.* **2015**, *32*, 2548–2558. [PubMed]

37. Shi, C.; Zhao, X.; Liu, Z.; Meng, R.; Chen, X.; Guo, N. Antimicrobial, antioxidant, and antitumor activity of epsilon-poly-L-lysine and citral, alone or in combination. *Food Nutr. Res.* **2016**, *60*, 31891–31898. [CrossRef] [PubMed]

38. Kim, S.H.; Bae, H.C.; Park, E.J.; Lee, C.R.; Kim, B.J.; Lee, S.; Park, H.H.; Kim, S.J.; So, I.; Kim, T.W.; et al. Geraniol inhibits prostate cancer growth by targeting cell cycle and apoptosis pathways. *Biochem. Biophys. Res. Commun.* **2011**, *407*, 129–134. [CrossRef] [PubMed]

39. Klein, G.; Rüben, C.; Upmann, M. Antimicrobial activity of essential oil components against potential food spoilage microorganisms. *Curr. Microbiol.* **2013**, *67*, 200–208. [CrossRef] [PubMed]

40. Tomazoni, E.Z.; Pansera, M.R.; Pauletti, G.F.; Moura, S.; Ribeiro, R.T.; Schwambach, J. In vitro antifungal activity of four chemotypes of *Lippia alba* (Verbenaceae) essential oils against *Alternaria solani* (Pleosporaceae) isolates. *An. Acad. Bras. Cienc.* **2016**, *31*, 999–1010. [CrossRef] [PubMed]

41. Anaruma, N.D.; Schmidt, F.L.; Duarte, M.C.; Figueira, G.M.; Delarmelina, C.; Benato, L.A.; Sartoratto, A. Control of *Colletotrichum gloeosporioides* (Penz.) Sacc. in yellow passion fruit using *Cymbopogon citratus* essential oil. *Braz. J. Microbiol.* **2010**, *41*, 66–73. [CrossRef] [PubMed]

42. Shukla, R.; Kumar, A.; Singh, P.; Dubey, N.K. Efficacy of *Lippia alba* (Mill.) N.E. Brown essential oil and its monoterpene aldehyde constituents against fungi isolated from some edible legume seeds and aflatoxin B1 production. *Int. J. Food Microbiol.* **2009**, *135*, 165–170. [CrossRef] [PubMed]

43. Singh, R.K. Fungitoxicity of some higher plants and synergistic activity of their essential oils against *Sclerotium rolfsii* Sacc. causing foot-rot disease of barley. *Hind. Antibiot. Bull.* **2005**, *47*, 45–51.

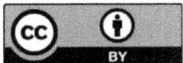

MDPI

Article

Antimicrobial, Cytotoxic, Phytotoxic and Antioxidant Potential of *Heliotropium strigosum* Willd.

Muhammad Khurm [1,*], Bashir A. Chaudhry [1], Muhammad Uzair [1] and Khalid H. Janbaz [2]

[1] Faculty of Pharmacy, Natural Product Chemistry Unit, Bahauddin Zakariya University, Multan 60800, Pakistan; drbashirahmadch@bzu.edu.pk (B.A.C.); muhammaduzair@bzu.edu.pk (M.U.)

[2] Akson College of Pharmacy, Mirpur University of Science and Technology, Mirpur 10250, Pakistan; KHjanbaz@hotmail.com

* Correspondence: khuram.ghori19@gmail.com; Tel.: +92-305-604-9669

Academic Editor: James D. Adams
Received: 26 May 2016; Accepted: 21 July 2016; Published: 28 July 2016

Abstract: Background: *Heliotropium strigosum* Willd. (Chitiphal) is a medicinally important herb that belongs to the *Boraginaceae* family. Traditionally, this plant was used in the medication therapy of various ailments in different populations of the world. The aim of the study is to probe the therapeutic aspects of *H. strigosum* described in the traditional folklore history of medicines. **Methods:** In the present study, the dichloromethane crude extract of this plant was screened to explore the antimicrobial, cytotoxic, phytotoxic and antioxidant potential of *H. strigosum*. For antibacterial, antifungal and antioxidant activities, microplate alamar blue assay (MABA), agar tube dilution method and diphenyl picryl hydrazine (DPPH) radical-scavenging assay were used, respectively. The cytotoxic and phytotoxic potential were demonstrated by using brine shrimp lethality bioassay and *Lemna minor* assay. **Results:** The crude extract displayed positive cytotoxic activity in the brine shrimp lethality assay, with 23 of 30 shrimps dying at the concentration of 1000 μg/mL. It also showed moderate phytotoxic potential with percent inhibition of 50% at the concentration of 1000 μg/mL. The crude extract exhibited no significant antibacterial activity against *Staphylococcus aureus*, *Shigella flexneri*, *Escherichia coli* and *Pseudomonas aeruginosa*. Non-significant antifungal and radical scavenging activity was also shown by the dichloromethane crude extract. **Conclusion:** It is recommended that scientists focus on the identification and isolation of beneficial bioactive constituents with the help of advanced scientific methodologies that seems to be helpful in the synthesis of new therapeutic agents of desired interest.

Keywords: *Heliotropium strigosum*; antimicrobial activity; cytotoxicity; phytotoxicity; antioxidant activity; *Boraginaceae* family

1. Introduction

For the past few decades, the importance of medicinal plants for treating various infections has been tremendously increased because of the fact that a large number of people belonging to different populations depend upon the usage of phytomedicines due to the unavailability of primary healthcare facilities [1]. According to World Health Organization reports on phytomedicines, more than 25% of drugs which have been prescribed in recent years are obtained from different plant sources [2]. The family *Boraginaceae* is comprised of 100 genera and about 2000 species. The plants of this family are widely distributed in temperate, especially Mediterranean and tropical, regions. In Pakistan, this family is represented by 32 genera and 135 species. Moreover, some species, namely *Cordia*, *Echium* and *Anchusa* are cultivated [3]. *Heliotropium*, *Cordia*, *Arnebia*, *Martensia* and *Trichodesma* are the important genera of the *Boraginaceae* family. Fruits of *Cordia* are used as diaphoretic and sometimes as astringent [4]. The leaves and roots of *Trichodesma indicum* are effective against snake bites and urinary diseases and are used as a diuretic. The roots of this plant are also applied as a paste on swellings and joints and are used in dysentery in children [5]. Today, *Alkanna* (*Alkanna tinctoria*) root is used almost exclusively as a cosmetic dye. Orally, it has been used for diarrhea and gastric ulcers. Traditionally, *Alkanna* root has been used topically to treat skin wounds and diseases [6].

Heliotropium is one of the most complex and largest genera of the family *Boraginaceae*. In tropical and temperate regions, it was represented by 270–275 species while in Pakistan 23 species of this genus are present [3]. In folk medicinal history, species of genus *Heliotropium* have attained noticeable pharmacological importance. In Somalia, the pulp of roots of *H. aegyptiacum* was considered to be effective against scorpion stings and snake bites [7]. In India, the paste of the leaves of *H. indicum* was used for rheumatism [8]. In Mauritius, the decoction of whole plant of *H. amplexicaule* was used in the therapeutic management of coughs and fevers [9]. The variety of traditional medicinal uses of *H. strigosum* made it distinguishable among other species of genus *Heliotropium*. The powder and decoction of the whole plant material of *H. strigosum* has been used in the medication therapy of rheumatic arthritis and jaundice and it is also used as a blood purifier [10]. The paste of roots of this plant is used for healing wounds [11]. For the curing of snake bites, gum boils, eye sores and nettle stings, the juice of this whole plant is administered [12]. This juice has also been used as diuretic and demonstrated some laxative effect [13]. In the current study, the dichloromethane crude extract of *H. strigosum* was examined for different biological activities, which could be related to the potential therapeutic value of this plant as prescribed in traditional medicine.

2. Experimental Section

2.1. Materials and Methods

The current study was conducted in the natural product chemistry laboratory, Faculty of Pharmacy, Bahauddin Zakariya University, new campus Multan and International Centre for Chemical and Biological Sciences, Hussain Ebrahim Jamal Research Institute of Chemistry, University of Karachi, Karachi, Pakistan, from August 2014 to August 2015.

2.2. Collection and Identification of Plant Material

The plant *Heliotropium strigosum* was collected in September 2014 from the surroundings of the railway ground district Khanewal (Pakistan) and identified by Dr. Muhammad Zafarullah, Assistant professor of Institute of Pure and Applied Biology, Bahauddin Zakariya University, Multan, Pakistan. A voucher no. "Stewart 591" was assigned to the specimen and preserved in the University herbarium.

2.3. Preparation of Dichloromethane Extract

Drying of the whole plant material was achieved by placing it under shade on old newspapers for 25 days to accomplish the process of effective extraction. When the plant material was completely dried, it was made into a coarse powder by crushing in the grinding mill. The extraction of this powdered plant material was carried out by the process of simple maceration. About 600 g of measured powdered material was put into the extraction bottle and a known volume of dichloromethane (3×1.5 L) was added into the bottle. For the purpose of maximum possible extraction, the mixture was continuously shaken after every 15 min for 3 to 4 h and then make it homogenized by the method of ultra-sonication. After 24 h, this mixture was filtered off. Repeated the same procedure thrice with dichloromethane. After the third collection, the dichloromethane extract was concentrated separately with the help of a rotary evaporator. This was done under reduced pressure. Then the dichloromethane extract was collected in the separated sample bottle and assigned the code as HSWPD (Heliotropium strigosum whole plant dichloromethane extract). The powdered plant material yielded 5.15 g of crude dichloromethane extract which is approximately 0.85% of total dry weight.

2.4. Antimicrobial Assays

2.4.1. Antibacterial Assay—Microplate Alamar Blue Assay (MABA)

The dichloromethane extract of *H. strigosum* was tested for significant antibacterial activity by using microplate alamar blue assay (MABA) (Invitrogen Corporation, San Diego, CA, USA). Strains of four pathogenic bacteria such as *Staphylococcus aureus* (NCTC 6571), *Shigella flexneri*, *Pseudomonas aeruginosa* (ATCC 10145) and *Escherichia coli* (NCTC 10418) were used in this assay. Mueller Hinton medium was prepared in a separate petri dish by following the specifications and guidelines given by the manufacturer (Sigma-Aldrich, St. Louis, MO, USA) and adjusted the pH to 6.6–7.3 normally at 25 °C. In this method, the tested micro-organisms were cultured in Mueller Hinton medium. Then the adjustment of turbidity index of inoculums up to 0.5 McFarland was done. We prepared the standard solution of 1g dichloromethane crude extract in 1 mL sterile dimethyl sulfoxide (DMSO) and distributed the above prepared media into the wells. This work was repeated thrice. All the tested micro-organisms were also placed into the wells. We made sure that the control wells did not contain any testing organism. The volume of well plate 96 was settled up to the level of 200 µL. At the end, added 5×10^6 cells into all the control and testing wells. Sealed all the plates with the help of paraffin. We placed these plates into the incubator at 37 °C for at least 18–20 h without shaking. After 20 h, we added 5 µL alamar blue dye into every well and shook gently at the speed of 80 revolutions per minute for 2–3 h by using the shaking incubator at 37 °C. Plates were covered with foil in shaking incubator. If the color of alamar blue dye was changed from blue to pink, it confirmed the growth of bacteria. Finally, the absorbance at the wavelength of 570 nm–600 nm was recorded with the help of Elisa reader [14].

2.4.2. Antifungal Assay—Agar Tube Dilution Method

The dichloromethane extract of whole plant of *H. strigosum* was tested for certain antifungal activity against six fungal strains such as *Trychophyton rubrum*, *Aspergillus niger*, *Fusarium solani*, *Candida albicans* and *Microsporum canis* by using agar tube dilution assay. We took 24 mg of dichloromethane crude extract and mixed in 1 mL sterile dimethyl sulfoxide (DMSO) to prepare its stock solution. For the preparation of Sabouraud dextrose agar (SDA) medium, we dissolved 32.5 g of Sabouraud glucose (2%) or maltose agar in 500 mL of distilled water. Adjusted the pH of this medium up to 5.5–5.6. Steaming of this media was done to dissolve all the suitable contents and added an appropriate volume (4 mL) into the test tubes having screw caps. These tubes were placed into the autoclave for 15 min at the temperature of 121 °C. After this, these tubes were placed at the temperature of 50 °C to achieve the effective cooling. Then, we loaded the non-solidified agar media by using pipette with 66.6 µL of tested sample taken from the stock solution. At room temperature, these tubes were placed for solidification in a slanting position. In every tube, a piece of fungus obtained from the seven day old fungus culture with the diameter of 4 mm was inoculated. All these tubes containing culture of fungus were placed in the incubator at the optimum temperature of 27 °C–29 °C. These culture containing tubes were allowed to grow for 3–7 days. This culture was observed twice a week during the period of incubation. When the incubation for 3–7 days was completed, the tube in which the growth of fungus culture was not visible was taken for the measurement of MIC value of the tested sample which is expressed in µg/mL [15].

2.5. Cytotoxic Assay—Brine Shrimp Lethality Bioassay

We stored the brine shrimp (*Artemia salina* Leach) eggs usually at the very low temperature of 4 °C. When filtration of brine solution was achieved, the hatching tray was filled half with this solution. Then we sprinkled eggs (50 mg) on the hatching try and incubated at the temperature of 37 °C. Then, we prepared the stock solution by taking 20 mg of crude dichloromethane extract and dissolved it in 2 mL of sterile dimethyl sulfoxide. From this stock solution, we transferred 5 µL, 50 µL and 500 µL into three separate glass vials at the concentrations of (10, 100 and 1000) µg/mL by using micro-pipette.

We placed these solvent containing vials over night for the evaporation of solvent. After two days of hatching process, we placed 10 larvae individually in the vials by using Pasteur pipette. We made the final volume of solvent up to 5 mL with the addition of sea water. These vials were placed into the incubator at the temperature of 25–27 °C for 24 h beneath the illumination. We took an extra two vials, one of which had the standard cytotoxic drug (Etoposide) served as positive control and the other vials in which respective solvent was added and served as negative control. Larvae were observed in each vial after 24 h. The number of survivors should be determined. Finney computerized system (Probit analysis) was used to analyze the data for the determination of LD_{50} values with 95% confidence intervals. Shrimps can be used 48–72 h after the initiation of hatching. After 72 h they should be discarded [15–17].

2.6. Phytotoxic Assay—Lemna Bioassay for Phytotoxicity

We prepared the inorganic E-medium (stock solution) by mixing appropriate inorganic constituents [15] into 1 liter of distilled water. The pH of E-medium was adjusted by adding potassium hydroxide pellets up to 6–7. To prepare the working E-medium, 100 mL of this stock solution was taken and dissolved it in 900 mL of distilled water. Then, we prepared the solution of tested crude extract by dissolving 30 mg of crude extract in 1.5 mL of ethyl alcohol. Three flasks were taken and pipetted 10 µL, 100 µL and 1000 µL into these flasks from concentration solutions of (10, 100 and 1000) µg/mL. Placed these solvent containing flasks over night for the evaporation of solvent. In each flask, added 20 mL stock solution of working E-medium along with the addition of 2 to 3 fronds (total fronds used 20) from the rosette of the plant *Lemna minor*. Two supplemented flasks, one with the standard drug (Paraquat) and other with the E-medium were served as positive and negative control respectively. We placed all these flasks into the growth chamber for 7 days by maintaining the temperature at 28 °C along with the light intensity of 9000 lux and relative humidity of 56% ± 10%. When the incubation period was completed, counted and verified the number of fronds of each flask on the 7th day [18,19]. The results which were analyzed as growth inhibition (%), compared with reference drug to negative control were given as shown below.

$$\% \text{ inhibition of growth } = 100 - (\text{No. of fronds in tested sample/No. of fronds in negative control}) \times 100$$

2.7. Antioxidant Assay—DPPH (2,2-Diphenyl-1-Picrylhydrazl) Radical Scavenging Assay

We dissolved the weighed amount of tested sample in a suitable volume of pure dimethyl sulfoxide. Then we prepared the 300 µL solution of DPPH (2,2-diphenyl-1-picrylhydrazl) by using appropriate volume of pure ethyl alcohol. About 5 µL of the tested sample solution was added into the 96-well plate and measured the absorbance at the wavelength of 515 nm. After this, to each well was added 95 µL solution of DPPH. We then incubated the 96 well plate at the temperature of 37 °C for the period of 30 min. We covered this plate with paraffin so that the solvent evaporation must be avoided. The pure dimethyl sulfoxide was served as control. By using a micro-plate reader, final absorbance at the wavelength of 515 nm was recorded. Percentage of radical scavenging activity (%RSA) can be determined by the following equation [20].

$$\% \text{ RSA } = 100 - (\text{Original dose of tested sample/Original dose of control}) \times 100$$

3. Results

3.1. Antibacterial Activity

In the present study, antibacterial potential of crude dichloromethane extract was examined. The percent (%) inhibition showed by sample extract against various tested bacteria are specified in the Table 1. The results of preliminary antibacterial activity demonstrated that the dichloromethane crude extract of *H. strigosum* showed inhibition up to 16% against *S. aureus* while against *S. flexneri*, and showed an inhibition of 3% respectively at the concentration used, which is 150 µg/mL. The pathogens *E. coli* and *P. aeruginosa* showed no inhibition against the tested sample. Thus, crude dichloromethane extract showed non-significant antibacterial activity against all the four tested bacterial strains when compared with the reference drug used, which was Ofloxacin (0.25 µg/mL).

Table 1. Results of preliminary antibacterial assay of *H. strigosum*.

Name of Bacteria	Percent (%) Inhibition of Tested Sample	Percent (%) Inhibition of Standard Drug (Ofloxacin)
S. aureus	16	92.35
E. coli	0	90.20
P. aeruginosa	0	89.35
S. flexneri	3	91.40

Concentration of tested sample used = 150 µg/mL; Concentration of standard drug used = 0.25 µg/mL; Positive control = Ofloxacin (standard antibiotic); Negative control = DMSO (Dimethyl sulfoxide); Percent inhibition activity, 0–39 = Low (non-significant); 40–59 = moderate; 60–69 = Good; above 70 = Significant.

3.2. Antifungal Activity

The dichloromethane extract of the whole plant of *H. strigosum* was tested for significant antifungal activity. The results shown by tested crude extract against different fungal strains are given in Table 2. The results revealed that none of the tested fungal strains showed any kind of inhibition against the tested sample. So, the dichloromethane extract was found to be inactive against all the tested fungus species at the concentration of the sample used (400 µg/mL).

Table 2. Results of antifungal assay of *H. strigosum*.

Name of Fungus	Linear Growth (mm)		% Inhibition (Tested Sample)	Standard Drug	MIC (µg/mL)
	Sample	Control			
T. rubrum	100	100	0	Miconazole	97.8
A. niger	100	100	0	Amphotericin B	20.70
F. solani	100	100	0	Miconazole	73.50
C. albicans	100	100	0	Miconazole	113.1
M. canis	100	100	0	Miconazole	98.1

MIC = Minimum inhibitory concentration; Concentration of tested sample used = 400 µg/mL; Percent inhibition activity, 0–39 = Low (non-significant); 40–59 = moderate; 60–69 = Good; above 70 = Significant; Positive control = Miconazole and Amphotericin B (*A. niger*); Negative control = DMSO (Dimethyl sulfoxide).

3.3. Cytotoxic Activity

Brine shrimp lethality bioassay was used for cytotoxic screening of dichloromethane extract of the whole plant of *H. strigosum*. The consequences of dichloromethane screening are expressed in Table 3. The results showed that, at the concentration of 10 µg/mL and 100 µg/mL, the number of dead shrimps was only one. However, when the concentration of the tested sample increased up to 1000 µg/mL, the number of dead shrimps was 23 and only 7 shrimps survived. Thus, from the above revealed data, an LD_{50} of 462 µg/mL was calculated as compared with the reference agent (etoposide) that resulted in an LD_{50} of 7.46 µg/mL.

Table 3. Results of brine shrimp lethality bioassay of *H. strigosum*.

Dose of Tested Sample (µg/mL)	No. of Shrimps	No. of Survivors	LD_{50} (µg/mL)	Standard Drug	LD_{50} (µg/mL)
10	30	29			
100	30	29	462	Etoposide	7.46
1000	30	7			

Positive control = Etoposide; Negative control = DMSO (Dimethyl sulfoxide); No. of replicates = 3; Incubation conditions = 28 ± 1 °C.

3.4. Phytotoxic Activity

The phytotoxic potential of dichloromethane extract of whole plant of *H. strigosum* was studied by using *Lemna minor* phytotoxicity bioassay. The growth inhibition (%) shown by the tested crude extract is given in Table 4. The results revealed that the tested sample showed percent growth inhibition up to 35% and 40% at the concentration of 10 and 100 μg/mL but at the concentration of 1000 μg/mL, it showed 50% growth inhibition. So, the dichloromethane extract exhibited low phytotoxic activity at the concentrations of 10 and 100 μg/mL but showed moderate activity at the highest tested concentration that was 1000 μg/mL when compared with the standard drug (Paraquat) which inhibited the growth of *L. minor* at the concentration of 0.015 μg/mL.

Table 4. Results of phytotoxicity assay of *H. strigosum*.

Name of Plant	Concentration of Tested Sample (μg/mL)	No. of Fronds		% Growth Inhibition	Concentration of Standard Drug (Paraquat) (μg/mL)
		Sample	Control		
Lemna minor	10	13		35	
	100	12	20	40	0.015
	1000	10		50	

Positive control = Paraquat; Negative control = Volatile solvent (ethanol); Incubation conditions = 28 ± 1 °C.

3.5. Antioxidant Activity

DPPH radical scavenging assay was used to determine the significant antioxidant activity of dichloromethane extract of the whole plant of *H. strigosum*. The radical scavenging activity exhibited by the tested dichloromethane extract is shown in Table 5. The results demonstrated that the crude extract showed non-significant antioxidant potential with very low radical scavenging activity up to 13% at the tested concentration that was 500 μM when compared with N-acetyl cysteine (standard drug) which exhibited significant radical scavenging activity up to 96% with IC_{50} of 111.44 ± 0.7 μM respectively at the same concentration.

Table 5. Results of diphenyl picryl hydrazine (DPPH) radical scavenging assay of *H. strigosum*.

Concentration of Tested Sample (μM)	% RSA (Radical Scavenging Activity)	$IC_{50} \pm SEM$ (μM)
500 [a]	13	>500
500 [b]	96	111.44 ± 0.7

[a] = Dichloromethane extract; [b] = N-acetyl cysteine (Standard drug & Positive control); Negative control = DMSO (Dimethyl sulfoxide); μM = Micro-molar (10^{-3} mol/m^3); SEM = Standard error mean; Data is expressed as mean $\pm$ SEM of three independent readings.

4. Discussion

The history of human beings has revealed that, for the past 60,000 years, plants have been used as a source of treating various ailments in different civilizations of the world [21]. Due to the increased resistance of microbes worldwide, scientists are always looking for the development of newer antibacterial agents [22]. Medicinal plants are considered as a source in the discovery and advancement of new pharmaceuticals which are effective in the management of different diseases [23,24]. In our study, the dichloromethane extract of whole plant material of *H. strigosum* showed non-significant antibacterial activity against *S. aureus*, *S. flexneri*, *E. coli* and *P. aeruginosa*. The results of our studies are quite comparable with the antibacterial activity revealed by other species of genus *Heliotropium* and some other plant species of different families. The petroleum ether and chloroform fractions of ethanolic extract of *H. subulatum* showed strong antibacterial activity against *E. coli*, *S. aureus*, *Streptococcus pneumonia* and *Bacillus subtilis*. That strong antibacterial activity might be due to the purification of five pyrrolizidine alkaloids from this plant [25]. The methaolic extract of aerial parts of *H. indicum* has broad spectrum antibacterial activity against *S. aureus*,

S. pneumonia, Salmonella typhi, E. coli and *Klebsiella pneumonia* [26]. The antibacterial significance of plant extracts is attributed mainly to the presence of terpenoids [27]. The sterols and triterpenoids such as β-sitosterol, stigmasterol, β-amyrin, friedelan-β-ol, cycloartenone, β-amyrin acetate and friedelin isolated from ethanol extract of the whole plant of *H. ellipticum* exhibited strong antibacterial activity against *E. coli, S. aureus* and *K. pneumonia* [28]. Filifolinol, one of the geranyl aromatic derivatives isolated from *H. sclerocarpum* and *H. filifolium* also showed significant antibacterial activity against *S. aureus, Bacillus cereus, B. subtilis* and *Micrococcus luteus* [29,30]. Another reported antibacterial potential was shown by the group of new 3 *H*-Spiro[1-benzofuran-2,1'-cyclohexane] derivatives such as 3'-hydroxy-2',2',6'-trimethyl-3*H*-spiro[1-benzofuran-2,1'-cyclohexane]-5-carboxylic acid, methyl 3'-acetyloxy-2',2',6'-trimethyl-3*H*-spiro[1-benzofuran-2,1'-cyclohexane]-5-carboxylate, methyl 3'-isopentanoyloxy-2',2',6'-trimethyl-3*H*-spiro[1-benzofuran-2,1'-cyclohexane]-5-carboxylate, and methyl 3'-benzoyloxy-2',2',6'-trimethyl-3*H*-spiro[1-benzofuran-2,1'-cyclohexane]-5-carboxylate isolated from the dichloromethane cuticle extract of *H. filifolium* against several gram positive and gram negative bacteria [31]. In addition to the genus *Heliotropium*, other plant species also exhibited antibacterial potential. The ethanolic extracts of *Curcuma longa* and *Alpinia galangal* displayed weak antibacterial activity against *S. aureus* and *S. typhi* and showed no inhibition against *B. subtilis, E. coli, P. aeruginosa* and *S. flexneri* [32]. Thus, from the above contributions, researchers have come to know that the identification, isolation and purification of different groups of organic compounds, mainly pyrrolizidine alkaloids, terpenoids and flavonoids, from *H. strigosum* should reveal that this plant has a perceptible future role in the field of antibacterial medicinal agents.

Different pathogenic fungi cause systemic infections of the skin, lungs, liver, mouth and blood [33–35]. Fungal attacks especially infect the skin and cause severe infections such as athlete's foot, tinea cruris and numerous others [36]. Only 10 antifungal drugs are permitted for the therapeutic management of invasive systemic fungal infections by the Food and Drug Administration (FDA) authority in United States of America [37]. Patients who have had pediatric lung transplantation are at serious risk of pulmonary fungal infection [33]. In the present study, the dichloromethane extract of whole plant material of *H. strigosum* demonstrated no antifungal activity and was found to be inactive against all the tested fungal strains. These results exposed the antifungal principles in a consistent manner, as established by different plant species of the family *Boraginaceae* and some other families. The methanolic extract of *Echium rauwolfii* and *E. horridum* showed no antifungal activity against *Aspergillus flavus* but were found to have weak activity against *C. albicans* [38]. The dichloromethane extract of *Cordia curassavica* [39] and *Cordia linnael* [40] showed equal antifungal activity to some extent against both *C. albicans* and *Clasdosporium cucumerinum*. The benzene extract of *Trichodesma amplexicaule* remained inactive against *Aspergillus niger* and *A. flavus* followed by chloroform extract with very low activity against these micro-organisms [41]. The ethyl acetate and n-butanol fractions of methanolic extract of *Onosma griffithii* reported no antifungal activity [42]. The ethyl alcohol and aqueous extracts of *Colendia procumbens* never showed antifungal activity against *C. albicans* [43]. No antifungal activity was displayed by the methanolic and aqueous extracts of *Trichodesma zeylanicum* and *Anchusa italic* [44]. Apart from the above consequences, different biological extracts and isolated bioactive constituents, mainly pyrrolizidine alkaloids and terpenoids from different *Heliotropium* species such as *H. indicum* [45], *H. ellipticum* [28,46] and *H. marifolium* [47], demonstrated significant antifungal activity against various pathogenic fungi. Our study reports for the first time the dichloromethane screening of *H. strigosum* for antifungal potential.

Due to the life threatening effects of cancer, it is known as a critical factors that increases the mortality rate worldwide. Cancer of the liver, lung, colon and stomach contribute to a major proportion of mortality cases all over the world [48]. In the present research work, the dichloromethane extract of *H. strigosum* shows positive cytotoxic activity with an LD_{50} of 462 μg/mL. The cytotoxic potential of this plant is extremely compatible with the previously reported developments in the field of antitumor drug discovery. The ethanolic, dichloromethane and n-hexane extracts of *H. subulatum* [49] and the methanolic extract of *H. indicum* [50] showed significant antineoplastic activity in the dose dependent manner. The ethanolic extracts of *Curcuma longa* and *Alpinia galangal* revealed strong cytotoxic potential with the LD_{50} of 33 $\mu g/mL$ and 109 $\mu g/mL$, respectively [32]. The occurrence of cytotoxic activity was mainly due to the presence of different classes of organic compounds such as phenolic compounds (polyphenols), catechins and flavonoid constituents. A large number of polyphenols and flavonoids have been purified and isolated from different parts of *Bruguiera gymnorrhiza*, *Blumea lacera*, *Aegiceras corniculatum*, *Hygrophila auriculata* and *Hibiscus tiliaceous*, which might be responsible for their cytotoxic activity. In 2007, a scientific report from Bangladesh examined 32 extracts of 16 different Bangladehsi plant species for their cytotoxic potential. Among these tested extracts, the aqueous extracts possessed very low cytotoxic potential. This low antitumor potential of aqueous extracts is of great therapeutic significance because traditionally they are used in the medication of various ailments instead of cancer [51]. Another informative description of cytotoxic potential was reported in Brazil in which 60 species of different medicinal plants were screened to examine the cytotoxic activity. Only 10% of plant species showed better cytotoxicity with ED_{50} less than 1000 ppm [16]. In most of the reported statistical data about the cytotoxic potential of different medicinal plants, scientists used brine shrimp lethality bioassay instead of other scientific approaches because a progressive correlation existed between the toxicity of brine shrimp and human nasopharyngeal carcinoma [52].

In the developing countries, weeds are considered an important factor for environmental protection. Approximately 30,000 different species of weeds are present in the world, out of which a reported 1800 cause the loss of 9.7% of crop yields [53]. The presence of weeds reduced the agricultural productivity of crops that lead to massive economical loss among different regions of the world. In a recent study, the dichloromethane extract of *H. strigosum* demonstrated moderate phytotoxic activity at the higher tested concentration (1000 $\mu g/mL$) but showed low phytotoxic activity at the concentration of 10 and 100 $\mu g/mL$ with the growth inhibition of 35% and 40%. The phytotoxic significances of this plant are followed by some other species of genus *Heliotropium* such as *H. dasycarpum* whose methanol and dichloromethane extract showed 100% inhibitory effect at the concentration of 1000 $\mu g/mL$, respectively [54]. Similar phytotoxic measurements were shown by ethanolic extract of *Curcuma longa* and *Alpinia galangal* [32]. The methanolic extract of *polygonatum verticillatum* exhibited significant phytotoxic activity at the tested doses of 5, 50 and 500 $\mu g/mL$ [55]. A few scientific descriptions of allelopathic approaches of *H. indicum* [56] and *Chrysanthemum morifolium* [57] were also considered. The reduction of crops quantity and quality is given serious attention by the scientists who focus upon the discovery and development of newer weedicides because chemically synthetic weedicides cause harmful adverse effects, mainly the expansion of weedicide resistant populations, lowering the water and soil consumption and resulting in damaging effects on non-targeted organisms [53].

The destructive effects of free radicals can be prevented by using different organic and inorganic substances having low molecular weight. Some of the commonly used antioxidative agents are tocopherols, copper, vitamin C, zinc, thiols, iron and manganese [58]. The recent scientific studies also exposed the beneficial preventive effects of antioxidants in the treatment of cardiovascular diseases, ocular damage and certain type of cancers [59]. The consequences of our study shows that the dichloromethane extract of *H. strigosum* demonstrated very low radical scavenging activity, only up to 13%. Therefore, no antioxidant activity was shown by the tested extract and it was found to be inactive. However, some other species of genus *Heliotropium* showed excellent radical scavenging activity because of the presence of flavonoids. Flavonoids are the largest group of naturally occurring phenolic compounds and possessed some chemical and biological properties which are very helpful in the prevention of free radicals formation. Flavonoids are found to be ubiquitous in most of the plants growing in extreme conditions [60]. A new compound belonging to the group of flavanones named as Naringenin was identified and isolated from the resinous exudate of dichloromethane extract of *H. sclerocarpum* which displayed outstanding free radical scavenging activity [30]. In 2009, from the resinous exudates of dichloromethane extract of *H. taltalense*, three flavonoids, namely Naringenin, 3-O-methylgalangin and 7-O-methyleriodictiol were isolated and exhibited significant antioxidant activity [61]. The isolation of three new flavonoids, namely, 5,3'-dihydroxy-7,4'-dimethoxyflavanone,

5,4′-dihydroxy-7-methoxyflavanone and 4′-acetyl-5-hydroxy-7-methoxyflavanone from *H. glutinosum* was also reported [60]. From *H. sinuatum*, eight previously reported flavonoids along with one new compound 4-(3′,5′-dihydroxynonadecyl) phenol were isolated, which confirmed the antioxidant behavior of this plant [62]. All the above previous scientific reports confirmed that all these plants showed exceptional antioxidant potential. This gives scientists a new approach to identify, purify and isolate the flavonoids and other phenolic compounds from *H. strigosum* which lead towards the synthesis of new antioxidant agents in the world of medicines.

5. Conclusions

The dichloromethane screening of *Heliotropium strigosum* was done for the first time. The crude extract of this plant showed low antibacterial activity against two bacterial stains, one is gram positive and other is gram negative. There was no antifungal activity shown by the tested crude extract. The dichloromethane extract exhibited positive cytotoxic and moderate phytotoxic potential at the highest tested concentrations. No antioxidant behavior was exposed by this plant. In conclusion, scientists and pharmacologists should pay serious attention to the screening of this plant by using some other scientific bioassay methodologies which might serve as a source for the identification, purification and isolation of beneficial bioactive constituents that seems to be helpful in the synthesis of new therapeutic agents of desired interest. Therefore, in the future, *Heliotropium strigosum* will be used globally as a source of safer phytomedicines.

Acknowledgments: We shall be very thankful to the management of Faculty of Pharmacy, Bahauddin Zakariya University, Multan and International Center for Chemical and Biological Sciences, Hussain Ebrahim Jamal Research Institute of Chemistry for providing us the necessary resources to perform these studies.

Author Contributions: Bashir Ahmed Chaudhry and Muhammad Uzair conceived and designed the project. Muhammad Khurm collected the plant material, performed the experiments and wrote the manuscript. Khalid Hussain Janbaz analyze the results and made the necessary corrections.

Conflicts of Interest: The authors declare no conflict of interest.

References

1.   Shanmugam, S.; Bhavani, P. Studies on the comparison of phytochemical constituents and antimicrobial activity of *Curcuma longa* varieties. *Int. J. Curr. Microbiol. Appl. Sci.* **2014**, *3*, 573–581.

2.   Pranuthi, E.K.; Narendra, K.; Swathi, J.; Sowjanya, K.; Reddi, K.R.; Emmanuel, R.F.S.; Satya, A.K. Qualitative Assessment of Bioactive Compounds from a Very Rare Medicinal Plant *Ficus dalhousiae* Miq. *J. Pharmacogn. Phytochem.* **2014**, *3*, 57–61.

3.   Nasir, E.; Ali, S. *Flora of West Pakistan*, 4th ed.; Feroz Sons Press: Karachi, Pakistan, 1974; p. 23.

4.   Ghori, M.K.; Ghaffarı, M.A.; Hussaın, S.N.; Manzoor, M.; Azız, M.; Sarwer, W. Ethnopharmacological, phytochemical and pharmacognostic potential of genus *Heliotropium* L. *Turk. J. Pharm. Sci.* **2016**, *13*, 143–168. [CrossRef]

5.   Shinwari, M.I.; Khan, M.A. Folk use of medicinal herbs of Margalla hills national park, Islamabad. *J. Ethnopharmacol.* **2000**, *69*, 45–56. [CrossRef]

6.   Bisset, N.G. *Max Wichtl's Herbal Drugs & Phytopharmaceuticals*; CRC Press: Boca Raton, FL, USA, 1994.

7.   Thulin, M. *Flora of Somalia*; CRB Press: Harare, NY, USA, 1993; Volume 1.

8.   Nagaraju, N.; Rao, K. A survey of plant crude drugs of Rayalaseema, Andhra Pradesh, India. *J. Ethnopharmacol.* **1990**, *29*, 137–158. [CrossRef]

9.   Schmelzer, G.; Gurib-Fakim, A. *Plant Resources of Tropical Africa*; Backurys Publishers: Leiden, The Netherlands, 2008; Volume 11.

10. Ahmad, S.; Alam, K.; Wariss, H.; Anjum, S.; Mukhtar, M. Ethnobotanical studies of plant resources of Cholistan desert, Pakistan. *Int. J. Sci. Res.* **2014**, *3*, 1782–1788.

11. Watanabe, T.; Rajbhandari, K.R.; Malla, K.J.; Yahara, S. *A Hand Book of Medicinal Plants of Nepal*; Kobfai Publishing Project: Bangkok, Thailand, 2005; Volume 15.

12. Roeder, E.; Wiedenfeld, H. Pyrrolizidine alkaloids in medicinal plants of Mongolia, Nepal and Tibet. *Die Pharm. Int. J. Pharm. Sci.* **2009**, *64*, 699–716.

13. Mahmood, A.; Mahmood, A.; Shaheen, H.; Qureshi, R.A.; Sangi, Y.; Gilani, S.A. Ethno medicinal survey of plants from district Bhimber Azad Jammu and Kashmir, Pakistan. *J. Med. Plants Res.* **2011**, *5*, 2348–2360.
14. Pettit, R.K.; Weber, C.A.; Kean, M.J.; Hoffmann, H.; Pettit, G.R.; Tan, R.; Horton, M.L. Microplate Alamar blue assay for *Staphylococcus epidermidis* biofilm susceptibility testing. *Antimicrob. Agents Chemother.* **2005**, *49*, 2612–2617. [CrossRef] [PubMed]
15. Atta-ur-Rahman; Choudhary, M.I.; William, J.T. *Bioassay Techniques for Drug Development*; CRC Press: Reading, UK, 2001; pp. 8–23.
16. Alves, T.M.D.A.; Silva, A.F.; Brandao, M.; Grandi, T.S.M.; Smania, E.D.F.A.; Smania, J. Biological screening of Brazilian medicinal plants. *Mem. Inst. Oswaldo Cruz* **2000**, *95*, 367–373. [CrossRef] [PubMed]
17. Mayer, B.N.; Ferrigni, N.R.; Putnam, J.E.; Jacobsen, L.B.; Nicholas, P.E.; McLaughlin, J.L. Brine Shrimp: A convenient general bioassay for active plant constituents. *Planta Med.* **1982**, *45*, 31–34. [CrossRef] [PubMed]
18. Atta-ur-Rehman. *Studies in Natural Product Chemistry*; Elsevier Science Publishers: Amsterdam, The Netherlands, 1991; Volume 9, pp. 383–409.
19. Rashid, R.; Farah, M.; Mirza, M.N. Biological screening of *Salvia cabulica*. *Pak. J. Bot.* **2009**, *41*, 1453–1462.
20. Uddin, N.; Siddiqui, B.S.; Begum, S.; Bhatti, H.A.; Khan, A.; Parveen, S.; Choudhary, M.I. Bioactive flavonoids from the leaves of *Lawsonia alba* (Henna). *Phytochem. Lett.* **2011**, *4*, 454–458. [CrossRef]
21. Sumner, J. *The Natural History of Medicinal Plants*; Timber Press: Portland, OR, USA, 2000; Volume 1.
22. Ullah, F.; Malik, S.; Ahmed, J. Antibiotic susceptibility pattern and ESBL prevalence in nosocomial *Escherichia coli* from urinary tract infections in Pakistan. *Afr. J. Biotechnol.* **2009**, *8*, 3921–3926.
23. Rafie, S.; MacDougall, C.; James, C.L. Cethromycin: A promising new ketolide antibiotic for respiratory infections. *Pharmacother.: J. Hum. Pharmacol. Drug Ther.* **2010**, *30*, 290–303. [CrossRef] [PubMed]
24. Angeh, J.E.; Huang, X.; Sattler, I.; Swan, G.E.; Dahse, H.; Härtl, A.; Eloff, J.N. Antimicrobial and anti-inflammatory activity of four known and one new triterpenoid from *Combretum imberbe* (Combretaceae). *J. Ethnopharmacol.* **2007**, *110*, 56–60. [CrossRef] [PubMed]
25. Singh, B.; Sahu, P.; Singh, S. Antimicrobial activity of pyrrolizidine alkaloids from *Heliotropium subulatum*. *Fitoterapia* **2002**, *73*, 153–155. [CrossRef]
26. Oluwatoyin, S.M.; Illeogbulam, N.G.; Joseph, A. Phytochemical and antimicrobial studies on the aerial parts of *Heliotropium indicum* Linn. *Ann. Biol. Res.* **2011**, *2*, 129–136.
27. Urzúa, A.; Rezende, M.C.; Mascayano, C.; Vásquez, L. A structure-activity study of antibacterial diterpenoids. *Molecules* **2008**, *13*, 882–891. [CrossRef] [PubMed]
28. Jain, S.; Singh, B.; Jain, R. Antimicrobial activity of triterpenoids from *Heliotropium ellipticum*. *Fitoterapia* **2001**, *72*, 666–668. [CrossRef]
29. Torres, R.; Villarroel, L.; Urzua, A.; Delle-Monache, F.; Delle-Monache, G.; Gacs-Baitz, E. Filifolinol, a rearranged geranyl aromatic derivative from the resinous exudate of *Heliotropium filifolium*. *Phytochemistry* **1994**, *36*, 249–250. [CrossRef]
30. Modak, B.; Salina, M.; Rodilla, J.; Torres, R. Study of the chemical composition of the resinous exudate isolated from *Heliotropium sclerocarpum* and evaluation of the antioxidant properties of the phenolic compounds and the resin. *Molecules* **2009**, *14*, 4625–4633. [CrossRef] [PubMed]
31. Urzúa, A.; Echeverría, J.; Rezende, M.C.; Wilkens, M. Antibacterial Properties of 3 H-Spiro [1-benzofuran-2, 1′-cyclohexane] Derivatives from *Heliotropium filifolium*. *Molecules* **2008**, *13*, 2385–2393. [CrossRef] [PubMed]
32. Khattak, S.; Shah, H.U.; Ahmad, W.; Ahmad, M. Biological effects of indigenous medicinal plants *Curcuma longa* and *Alpinia galanga*. *Fitoterapia* **2005**, *76*, 254–257. [CrossRef] [PubMed]
33. Danziger-Isakov, L.A.; Worley, S.; Arrigain, S.; Aurora, P.; Ballmann, M.; Boyer, D.; Conrad, C.; Eichler, I.; Elidemir, O.; Goldfarb, S. Increased mortality after pulmonary fungal infection within the first year after pediatric lung transplantation. *J. Heart Lung Transplant.* **2008**, *27*, 655–661. [CrossRef] [PubMed]
34. Fung, J.J. Fungal infection in liver transplantation. *Transpl. Infect. Dis.* **2002**, *4*, 18–23. [CrossRef] [PubMed]
35. Ker, C.C.; Hung, C.C.; Huang, S.Y.; Chen, M.; Hsieh, S.; Lin, C.; Chang, S.; Luh, K. Comparison of bone marrow studies with blood culture for etiological diagnosis of disseminated mycobacterial and fungal infection in patients with acquired immunodeficiency syndrome. *J. Microbiol. Immunol. Infect.* **2002**, *35*, 89–93. [PubMed]
36. Al-Sogair, S.; Moawad, M.; Al-Humaidan, Y. Fungal infection as a cause of skin disease in the eastern province of Saudi Arabia: Cutaneous candidosis. *Mycoses* **1991**, *34*, 429–431. [CrossRef] [PubMed]

37. Dismukes, W.E. Introduction to antifungal drugs. *Clin. Infect. Dis.* **2000**, *30*, 653–657. [CrossRef] [PubMed]

38. El-Shazly, A.; Abdel-All, M.; Tei, A.; Wink, M. Pyrrolizidine alkaloids from *Echium rauwolfii* and *Echium horridum* (*Boraginaceae*). *Z. Naturforschung. C J. Biosci.* **1999**, *54*, 295–300. [CrossRef]

39. Ioset, J.R.; Marston, A.; Gupta, M.P.; Hostettmann, K. Antifungal and larvicidal cordiaquinones from the roots of *Cordia curassavica*. *Phytochemistry* **2000**, *53*, 613–617. [CrossRef]

40. Ioset, J.R.; Marston, A.; Gupta, M.P.; Hostettmann, K. Antifungal and larvicidal meroterpenoid naphthoquinones and a naphthoxirene from the roots of *Cordia linnael*. *Phytochemistry* **1998**, *47*, 729–734. [CrossRef]

41. Singh, B.; Singh, S. Antimicrobial activity of terpenoids from *Trichodesma amplexicaule* Roth. *Phytother. Res.* **2003**, *17*, 814–816. [CrossRef] [PubMed]

42. Ahmad, B.; Ali, N.; Bashir, S.; Choudhary, M.I.; Azam, S.; Khan, I. Parasiticidal, antifungal and antibacterial activities of *Onosma griffithii* Vatke. *Afr. J. Biotechnol.* **2009**, *8*, 5084–5087.

43. Ramakrishnan, G.; Kothai, R.; Jaykar, B.; Rathnakumar, T.V. In vitro Antibacterial Activity of different extracts of Leaves of *Coldenia procumbens*. *Int. J. Pharm. Tech. Res.* **2011**, *3*, 1000–1004.

44. Bahraminejad, S. In vitro and in vivo antifungal activities of Iranian plant species against *Pythium aphanidermatum*. *Ann. Biol. Res.* **2012**, *3*, 2134–2143.

45. Rao, P.R.; Nammi, S.; Raju, A.D.V. Studies on the antimicrobial activity of *Heliotropium indicum* Linn. *J. Nat. Rem.* **2002**, *2*, 195–198.

46. Jain, S.C.; Sharma, R. Antimicrobial activity of pyrrolizidine alkaloids from *Heliotropium ellipticum*. *Chem. Pharm. Bull.* **1987**, *35*, 3487–3489. [CrossRef] [PubMed]

47. Singh, B.; Dubey, M. Estimation of triterpenoids from *Heliotropium marifolium* Koen. ex Retz. in vivo and in vitro. I. Antimicrobial screening. *Phytother. Res.* **2001**, *15*, 231–234. [CrossRef] [PubMed]

48. Das, S.; Das, M.K.; Mazumder, P.M.; Das, S.; Basu, S.P. Cytotoxic activity of methanolic extract of *Berberis aristata* DC. on colon cancer. *Glob. J. Pharmacol.* **2009**, *3*, 137–140.

49. Singh, B.; Sahu, P.; Jain, S.; Singh, S. Antineoplastic and antiviral screening of pyrrolizidine alkaloids from *Heliotropium subulatum*. *Pharm. Biol.* **2002**, *40*, 581–586. [CrossRef]

50. Rahman, M.A.; Mia, M.A.; Shahid, I.Z. Pharmacological and phytochemical screen activities of roots of *Heliotropium indicum* Linn. *Pharmacologyonline* **2011**, *1*, 185–192.

51. Uddin, S.J.; Grice, I.D.; Tiralongo, E. Cytotoxic effects of Bangladeshi medicinal plant extracts. *Evid. Based Complement. Altern. Med.* **2011**, *2011*, 1–7. [CrossRef] [PubMed]

52. Ateeq, R.; Mannan, A.; Inayatullah, S.; Akhtar, M.Z.; Qayyum, M.; Mirza, B. Biological evaluation of wild thyme (*Thymus serpyllum*). *Pharm. Biol.* **2009**, *47*, 628–633.

53. Li, Y.; Sun, Z.; Zhuang, X.; Xu, L.; Chen, S.; Li, M. Research progress on microbial herbicides. *Crop Prot.* **2003**, *22*, 247–252. [CrossRef]

54. Ghaffari, M.A.; Bano, S.; Hayat, K. Antimicrobial and Phytotoxic Effects of the Plant *Heliotropium Dasycarpum* L. *Int. J. Pharm. Biol. Sci.* **2013**, *4*, 339–345.

55. Saeed, M.; Khan, H.; Khan, M.A.; Simjee, S.U.; Muhammad, N.; Khan, S.A. Phytotoxic, insecticidal and leishmanicidal activities of aerial parts of *Polygonatum verticillatum*. *Afr. J. Biotechnol.* **2010**, *9*, 1241–1244.

56. Mongelli, E.; Desmarchelier, C.; Coussio, J.; Ciccia, G. The potential effects of allelopathic mechanisms on plant species diversity and distribution determined by the wheat rootlet growth inhibition bioassay in South American plants. *Rev. Chil. Hist. Nat.* **1997**, *70*, 83–89.

57. Beninger, C.W.; Hall, J.C. Allelopathic activity of luteolin 7-*O*-β-glucuronide isolated from *Chrysanthemum morifolium* L. *Biochem. Sys. Ecol.* **2005**, *33*, 103–111. [CrossRef]

58. Machlin, L.J.; Bendich, A. Free radical tissue damage: Protective role of antioxidant nutrients. *FASEB J.* **1987**, *1*, 441–445. [PubMed]

59. Stanner, S.A.; Hughes, J.; Kelly, C.N.M.; Buttriss, J. A review of the epidemiological evidence for the 'antioxidant hypothesis'. *Public Health Nutr.* **2004**, *7*, 407–422. [CrossRef] [PubMed]

60. Modak, B.; Rojas, M.; Torres, R.; Rodilla, J.; Luebert, F. Antioxidant activity of a new aromatic geranyl derivative of the resinous exudates from *Heliotropium glutinosum* Phil. *Molecules* **2007**, *12*, 1057–1063. [CrossRef] [PubMed]

61. Modak, B.; Rojas, M.; Torres, R. Chemical analysis of the resinous exudate isolated from *Heliotropium taltalense* and evaluation of the antioxidant activity of the phenolics components and the resin in homogeneous and heterogeneous systems. *Molecules* **2009**, *14*, 1980–1989. [CrossRef] [PubMed]
62. Modak, B.; Torres, R.; Lissi, E.; Monache, F.D. Antioxidant capacity of flavonoids and a new arylphenol of the resinous exudate from *Heliotropium sinuatum*. *Nat. Prod. Res.* **2003**, *17*, 403–407. [CrossRef] [PubMed]

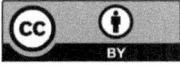

MDPI

Article

Heteromeles Arbutifolia, a Traditional Treatment for Alzheimer's Disease, Phytochemistry and Safety

Xiaogang Wang [1], Raphael Dubois [2], Caitlyn Young [2], Eric J. Lien [2] and James D. Adams [2,*]

[1] Tongji School of Pharmacy, Huazhong University of Science and Technology, Wuhan 430030, Hubei, China; wxg0122@163.com

[2] Department of Pharmacology and Pharmaceutical Sciences, School of Pharmacy, University of Southern California, Los Angeles, CA 90899-9121, USA; rd_820@usc.edu (R.D.); caitlyny@usc.edu (C.Y.); elien@usc.edu (E.J.L.)

* Correspondence: jadams@usc.edu; Tel.: +1-323-442-1362; Fax: +1-323-442-1681

Academic Editor: Gerhard Litscher
Received: 8 June 2016; Accepted: 27 June 2016; Published: 7 July 2016

Abstract: Background: This study examined the chemistry and safety of *Heteromeles arbutifolia*, also called toyon or California holly, which is a traditional California Indian food and treatment for Alzheimer's disease. **Methods:** Plant extracts were examined by HPLC/MS, NMR and other techniques to identify compounds. Volunteers were recruited to examine the acute safety of the plant medicine using a standard short-term memory test. **Results:** The plant was found to contain icariside E4, dihydroxyoleanenoic acid, maslinic acid, betulin, trihydroxyoxo-seco-ursdienoic acid, catechin, vicenin-2, farrerol, kaempferide and tetrahydroxyoleanenoic acid. These compounds are anti-inflammatory agents that may protect the blood-brain barrier and prevent inflammatory cell infiltration into the brain. The dried berries were ingested by six volunteers to demonstrate the safety of the medicine. **Conclusion:** The plant medicine was found to contain several compounds that may be of interest in the treatment of Alzheimer's disease. The plant medicine was found to be safe.

Keywords: *Heteromeles arbutifolia*; toyon; California holly; Alzheimer's disease; phytochemistry; safety

1. Introduction

Senile dementia, now commonly called Alzheimer's disease or vascular dementia, was known among California Indians before Europeans came to California [1]. The condition was commonly treated with a native plant, *Heteromeles arbutifolia*, also called toyon or California holly. The medicine consists of about 5 g of the dried berries which are slowly chewed and swallowed by the patient. The medicine slows down the progression of the disease and helps patients continue to have productive lives. The phytochemistry of the plant has not been adequately addressed, except for two publications that found cyanide in the plant [2,3]. There are reports of cyanide poisoning in insects and goats foraging on the leaves of the plant [3,4]. This indicates that the leaves of the plant may be toxic to some animal species. Most fruits from plants in the Rosaceae family contain cyanide, including apples, apricots, peaches, cherries and plums. The berries of *H. arbutifolia* are eaten fresh and cooked as foods by California Indians and other people [1]. The current study examined the chemistry and safety of the plant medicine.

Several plant-derived compounds are known to be protective in models of Alzheimer's disease, including flavonoids, resveratrol, green tea polyphenols, curcumin and ferulic acid [5–9]. Ferulic acid is an antioxidant derived from fruits, vegetables and grains. It prevents beta-amyloid fibril formation and is neuroprotective.

2. Experimental Section

Plant material: The leaves of *H. arbutifolia* were collected in May in a canyon near Pasadena, CA, USA, and were used for phytochemical analysis. The fruit of the plant were collected in October in the same location and were made into the plant medicine. The leaves were stored frozen. The fruit were dehydrated with a food dehydrator and stored frozen.

Preparation of solvent extraction and isolation: The frozen leaves (123 g) were thawed and added to 275 mL of ultrapure water, finely chopped with a blender and extracted with 500 mL of ultrapure acetonitrile to make a preparation for phytochemical analysis. Column chromatography was performed with Silicagel 60 columns (EMD, Darmstadt, Germany) that were developed with the following solvents: ethyl acetate (20%, 30%, then 100%) in hexane. Six fractions were collected and checked by analytical TLC using 20% ethyl acetate in hexane. The plates were sprayed with 10% sulfuric acid and heated to visualize spots. Column purified fractions were further purified by preparative TLC (250 μm thick plates, EMD, Darmstadt, Germany) in 20% or 30% ethyl acetate/hexane. Several bands were scraped from each preparative TLC plate. Some bands were further purified by preparative TLC.

NMR spectra (^{1}H and ^{13}C NMR) were recorded at room temperature with a Varian Mercury Plus instrument at 400 MHz. Chemical shifts (δ) are reported in ppm relative to TMS. HPLC/MS analysis involved a Thermo Finnigan LCQ DECA (Waltham, MA, USA) with a reverse phase column. The solvent system consisted of 10% MeOH in water that increased at 2% per min to 100% MeOH.

Volunteers were recruited from the community by word of mouth and posters. Each volunteer claimed to be of normal health and no history of dementia. All six volunteers were male and ranged from 21 to 60 years old. Each volunteer was administered the modified mini-mental state test [10], which is routinely used to assess Alzheimer's disease in patients. They then chewed and swallowed 5 g of the dried berries. After 30 min, they were again administered the mini-mental state test. Each volunteer served as their own control since they were examined before and after ingesting the medicine. There was no blinding of the subjects or investigators, since the purpose was to examine the safety of the medicine.

This work was performed in accordance with the Declaration of Helsinki. Each volunteer signed an informed consent document. All personal information on each volunteer was kept confidential.

3. Results

Several known compounds were identified in the plant extract by HPLC/MS, UV and NMR. Despite reports of cyanide in the leaves of the plant, no cyanogenic compounds were found. The identified compounds were all known compounds. Data for each compound matched published data: icariside E4 [11], 2A,3β-dihdroxyolean 13(18)-en-28-oic acid [12], maslinic acid [13–15], betulin [16,17], trihydroxy19-oxo-18,19-seco-urs-11,13(18)-dien-28-oic acid [12], catechin [18], vicenin-2 [18], farrerol [19,20], kaempferide [21], 2A,3α,19α,23-tetrahydroxyolean-12-en-28-oic acid [12], lupeol acetate [22]. The data found in this study are shown below.

3.1. Icariside E4

UV/Vis λmax (MeOH) nm (logε): 230, 280.

MS (CI, 70 eV): m/z (%) = 507 [M + H$^+$] (100).

2A,3β-Dihdroxyolean13(18)-en-28-oic acid.

UV/Vis λmax (MeOH) nm (logε): 235, 280.

MS (CI, 70 eV): m/z (%) = 495 [M + Na$^+$] (60), 391 (100), 383, 149.

3.2. Maslinic Acid

UV/Vis λmax (MeOH) nm (logε): 232, 275.

MS (EI, 70 eV): m/z (%) = 471 [M$^+$] (20), 419 (100).

3.3. Betulin

UV/Vis λmax (MeOH) nm (logε): 235, 265.

^{1}H NMR (400 MHz, CDCl3): 0.89, 1.66 (2H, m, CH2), 1.52, 1.57 (2H, m, CH2), 3.0 (1H, m, CH), 1.07 (1H, m, CH), 1.34, 1.47 (2H, m, CH2), 1.36, 1.42 (2H, m CH2), 1.11 (1H, m, CH), 1.21, 1.45 (2H, m, CH2), 1.48, 1.51 (2H, m, CH2), 1.67 (1H, s, CH), 1.07, 1.7 (2H, m, CH2), 1.23, 1.92 (2H, m, CH2), 1.32 (1H, m, CH), 2.2 (1H, m, CH), 1.4, 2.0 (2H, m, CH2), 1.06, 1.86 (2H, m, CH2), 0.96 (3H, s, Me), 0.75 (3H, s, Me), 0.81 (3H, s, Me), 0.91 (3H, s, Me), 0.96 (6H, s, 2Me), 3.2 (2H, m, CH2), 3.66 (3H, s, Me), 4.6, 4.75 (2H, d, CH2, J = 15 Hz).

^{13}C NMR (400 MHz, CDCl3): 12.3 (C23), 19.9 (C29), 20.3 (C26), 20.7 (C6), 20.9 (C11), 22.5 (C25), 23.3 (C24), 24.0 (C22), 26.5 (C2), 28.0 (C12), 28.7 (C15), 29.6 (C20), 30.2 (C16), 34.6 (C21), 34.9 (C7), 35.8 (C1), 38.1 (C4), 38.4 (C10), 39.0 (C13), 39.4 (C8), 41.4 (C14), 47.1 (C17), 47.8 (C18), 48.1 (C19), 48.8 (C9), 54.0 (C5), 68.3 (C27), 78.3 (C3), 110.4 (C30), 150.7 (C28).

MS (CI, 70 eV): m/z (%) = 443 [M+H$^+$] (50), 429 [MH-CH$_2$$^+$] (100).

Trihydroxy19-oxo-18,19-seco-urs-11,13(18)-dien-28oic acid.

UV/Vis λmax (MeOH) nm (logε): 240.

MS (CI, 70 eV): m/z (%) = 523 [M+Na$^+$], 501 [M+H$^+$], 439.

3.4. Catechin

UV/Vis λmax (MeOH) nm (logε): 240, 280.

MS (CI, 70 eV): m/z (%) = 291 [M+H$^+$], 161, 147, 139, 123.

3.5. Vicenin-2

UV/Vis λmax (MeOH) nm (logε): 230, 270, 340.

MS (EI, 70 eV): m/z (%) = 593 [M$^+$], 455, 358, 295

3.6. Farrerol

UV/Vis λmax (MeOH) nm (logε): 291, 337.

MS (CI, 70 eV): m/z (%) = 301 [M+H$^+$], 282, 152, 120.

3.7. Kaempferide

UV/Vis λmax (MeOH) nm (logε): 289, 337.

MS (EI, 70 eV): m/z (%) = 301 [M+H$^+$], 258, 210.

2A,3α,19α,23-Tetrahydroxyolean-12-en-28-oic acid.

UV/Vis λmax (MeOH) nm (logε): 233, 283.

MS (EI, 70 eV): m/z (%) = 503 [M$^-$], 451.

3.8. Lupeol Acetate

UV/Vis λmax (MeOH) nm (logε): 233, 399.

MS (EI, 70 eV): m/z (%) = 469 [M+H$^+$], 443, 425 [M-Ac], 409, 184.

The safety of the plant medicine was demonstrated in six volunteers. Each volunteer scored 100% on the modified mini-mental state test before and after ingesting 5 g of the berries. No volunteer complained of any adverse effects from eating the berries, which were reported to taste like sweet apples. There were no obvious signs of cyanide poisoning in any individual. The berries of the plant are a traditional food and medicine of California Indians [1].

4. Discussion

Several compounds that may be beneficial in the treatment of Alzheimer's disease were found. A recent paper suggests that Alzheimer's disease may be caused by damage to the blood-brain barrier which allows macrophages and other inflammatory cells to invade the brain and increase the formation of amyloid plaques and neurofibrillary tangles [23].

Icariside compounds, similar to icariside E4, were found in *H. arbutifolia* and are known to protect the blood-brain barrier, prevent the infiltration of inflammatory cells into the brain and prevent neuronal damage [19,24]. An unknown that is either maslinic acid [8–10] or pomolic acid [13,25] was found. Maslinic acid is well known to occur in plants in the Rosaceae family, whereas pomolic acid is not. This implies that the compound found in the current study is maslinic acid. Maslinic acid suppresses nuclear factor kappa B which decreases the secretion of tumor necrosis factor α by astrocytes [26]. This is an anti-inflammatory effect that protects the blood-brain barrier since tumor necrosis factor α is involved in stimulating the production of vascular endothelial adhesion factors that increase the adhesion and transmigration of inflammatory cells across the blood-brain barrier [27].

Flavonoids seem to be beneficial in the prevention of Alzheimer's disease [28]. Flavonoids such as catechin were found in the plant and stimulate the non-amyloidogenic cleavage of amyloid precursor protein. Vicenin-2 inhibits the glycation of proteins, an anti-inflammatory effect [29]. Farrerol protects the blood-brain barrier by inhibiting the destruction of endothelial cells through apoptosis [30]. Kaempferide is 4'-methylkaempferol. Kaempferol is neuroprotective in a model of Alzheimer's disease and reverses amyloid beta–induced neuronal impairment [31]. It remains to be shown if kampferide has similar actions.

Betulin was a major component in the plant and it prevents sterol regulatory element binding protein activation [32]. It improves insulin resistance and decreases fat build-up in atherosclerosis. By the inhibition of the sterol regulatory element binding protein, it inhibits genes involved in fat accumulation. This may prevent the accumulation of perivascular fat that secretes adipokines such as visfatin. Visfatin may be involved in damaging the blood-brain barrier in Alzheimer's disease [23].

Lupeol acetate was found in the plant and is a triterpene that has anti-inflammatory properties through the modulation of the brain opioid system and tumor necrosis factor α [33]. This is potentially useful in the treatment of Alzheimer's disease.

H. arbutifolia must not be confused with English holly, *Ilex aquifolium*. Although both plants have red berries and spiny leaves, *I. aquifolium* berries are poison, whereas *H. arbutifolia* berries are not.

5. Conclusions

The traditional medicine *H. arbutifolia* has a number of active compounds that are potentially beneficial in Alzheimer's disease. This plant medicine may provide new leads for drug therapy in the disease. The phytochemistry of the plant indicates that protection of the blood-brain barrier and prevention of inflammatory cell infiltration into the brain may be important targets in the treatment of Alzheimer's disease. It may be worthwhile to investigate the use of the plant medicine itself in Alzheimer's disease.

Acknowledgments: This work was supported by a Visiting Scholar Fellowship from the government of China awarded to Xiaogang Wang.

Author Contributions: All authors conceived and designed the experiments; Xiaogang Wang, Raphael Dubois, Caitlyn Young and James D. Adams performed the experiments; all authors analyzed the data; James D. Adams contributed reagents/materials/analysis tools; all authors contributed to writing the paper.

Conflicts of Interest: The authors declare no conflict of interest.

References

1. Garcia, C.; Adams, J. *Healing with Medicinal Plants of the West Cultural and Scientific Basis for Their Use*, 3rd ed.; Abedus Press: La Crescenta, CA, USA, 2012; pp. 123–125.
2. Dement, W.; Mooney, H. Seasonal variation in the production of tannins and cyanogenic glucosides in the chaparral shrub *Heteromeles arbutifolia*. *Oecologia* **1974**, *15*, 65–76. [CrossRef]
3. Dahlman, D.; Johnson, V. *Heteromeles arbutifolia* (Rosaceae: Pomoideae) found toxic to insects. *Entomol. News* **1980**, *91*, 141–142.
4. Teqzes, J.; Puschner, B.; Melton, L. Cyanide toxicosis in goats after ingestion of California Holly (*Heteromeles arbutifolia*). *J. Vet. Diagn. Investig.* **2003**, *15*, 478–480. [CrossRef]
5. Pocernich, C.; Lange, M.; Sultana, R.; Butterfield, D. Nutritional approaches to modulate oxidative stress in Alzheimer's disease. *Curr. Alzheimer Res.* **2011**, *8*, 452–469. [CrossRef] [PubMed]
6. Picone, P.; Bondi, M.; Montana, G.; Bruno, A.; Pitarresi, G.; Giammona, G.; di Carlo, M. Ferulic acid inhibits oxidative stress and cell death induced by Ab oligomers: Improved delivery by solid lipid nanoparticles. *Free. Radic. Res.* **2009**, *43*, 1133–1145. [CrossRef] [PubMed]
7. Ono, K.; Hirohata, M.; Yamada, M. Ferulic destabilizes preformed beta-amyloid fibrils in vitro. *Biochem. Biophys. Res. Commun.* **2005**, *336*, 444–449. [CrossRef] [PubMed]
8. Sgarbossa, A.; Giacomazza, D.; di Carlo, M. Ferulic acid: A hope for Alzheimer's disease therapy from plants. *Nutrients* **2015**, *7*, 5764–5782. [CrossRef] [PubMed]
9. Jung, J.; Yan, J.; Li, H.; Sultan, M.; Yu, J.; Lee, H.; Shin, K.; Song, D. Protective effects of a dimeric derivative of ferulic acid in animal models of Alzheimer's disease. *Eur. J. Pharmacol.* **2016**, *782*, 30–34. [CrossRef] [PubMed]
10. Teng, E.; Chui, H. The modified mini-mental state (3MS) examination. *J. Clin. Psychiatry* **1987**, *48*, 314–318. [PubMed]
11. Miyase, T. Ionone and lignan glycosides from *Epimedium diphyllum*. *Phytochemistry* **1989**, *28*, 3483–3485. [CrossRef]
12. Zeng, N.; Shen, Y.; Li, L.; Jiao, W.; Gao, P.; Song, S.; Chen, W.; Lin, H. Antiinflammatory triterpenes from the leaves of *Rosa laevigata*. *J. Nat. Prod.* **2011**, *74*, 732–738. [CrossRef] [PubMed]
13. Numata, A. Cytotoxic triterpenes from a Chinese medicine, Goreishii. *Chem. Pharm. Bull.* **1989**, *37*, 648–651. [CrossRef] [PubMed]
14. Hossain, M.; Ismail, Z. Isolation and characterization of triterpenes from the leaves of *Orthosiphon stamineus*. *Arab. J. Chem.* **2013**, *6*, 295–298. [CrossRef]
15. Chaudhuri, P.; Singh, D. A new triterpenoid from the rhizomes of *Nelumbo nucifera*. *Nat. Prod. Res.* **2013**, *27*, 532–536. [CrossRef] [PubMed]
16. Hayek, E.; Jordis, U.; Moche, W.; Sauter, F. A bicentennial of betulin. *Phytochemistry* **1989**, *28*, 2229–2242. [CrossRef]
17. Kim, D.; Chen, Z.; Nguyen, V.; Pezzuto, J.; Qiu, S.; Lu, Z. A concise semi-synthetic approach to betulinic acid from betulin. *Synth. Commun.* **1997**, *27*, 1607–1612. [CrossRef]
18. Grayer, R.; Kite, G.; Abou-Zaid, M.; Archer, L. The application of atmospheric pressure chemical ionization liquid chromatography-mass spectrometry in the chemotaxonomic study of flavonoids: Characterization of flavonoids from *Ocimum gratissimum* var. *gratissimum*. *Phytochem. Anal.* **2000**, *11*, 257–267. [CrossRef]
19. Youssef, D.; Ramadan, M.; Khalifa, A. Acetophenones, a chalcone, a chromone and flavonoids from *Pancratium maritimum*. *Phytochemistry* **1998**, *49*, 2579–2583. [CrossRef]
20. Iwashina, T.; Kitamjima, J.; Matsumoto, S. Flavonoids in the species of *Cyrtomium* (Dryopteridaceae) and related genera. *Biochem. Syst. Ecol.* **2006**, *34*, 14–24. [CrossRef]
21. Baracco, A.; Bertin, G.; Gnocco, E.; Legorati, M.; Sedocco, S.; Catinella, S.; Favretto, D.; Traldi, P. A comparison of the combination of fast-atom bombardment with tandem mass spectrometry and of gas chromatography with mass spectrometry in the analysis of a mixture of kaempferol, kaempferide, luteolin and oleuropein. *Rapid Commun. Mass Spectrom.* **1995**, *9*, 427–436. [CrossRef]
22. Saratha, V.; Pillai, I.; Subramanian, S. Isolation and characterization of lupeol, a triterpenoid from *Calotropis gigantea* latex. *Int. J. Pharm. Sci. Rev. Res.* **2011**, *10*, 54–57.

23. Adams, J. Alzheimer's disease, ceramide, visfatin and NAD. *CNS Neurol. Disord. Drug. Targets* **2008**, *7*, 492–498. [CrossRef]

24. Yan, B.; Pan, C.; Mao, X.; Yang, L.; Liu, Y.; Yan, L.; Mu, H.; Wang, C.; Sun, K.; Liao, F.; et al. Icariside II improves cerebral microcirculatory disturbance and alleviates hippocampal injury in gerbils after ischemia reperfusion. *Brain Res.* **2014**, *1573*, 63–73. [CrossRef] [PubMed]

25. Lee, T.; Juang, S.; Hsu, F.; Wu, S. Triterpene acids from the leaves of *Planchonella duclitan* (Blanco) Bakhuizan. *J. Chin. Chem. Soc.* **2005**, *52*, 1275–1280. [CrossRef]

26. Huang, L.; Guan, T.; Qian, Y.; Huang, M.; Tang, X.; Li, Y.; Sun, H. Anti-inflammatory effects of maslinic acid, a natural triterpene, in cultured cortical astrocytes via suppression of nuclear factor-kappa B. *Eur. J. Pharmacol.* **2011**, *672*, 169–174. [CrossRef] [PubMed]

27. Tak, P.; Taylor, P.; Breedveld, F.; Smeets, T.; Daha, M.; Kluin, P.; Meinders, A.; Maini, R. Decrease in cellularity and expression of adhesion molecules by anti-tumor necrosis factor α monoclonal antibody treatment in patients with rheumatoid arthritis. *Arthritis Rheum.* **1996**, *39*, 1077–1081. [CrossRef] [PubMed]

28. Mandel, S.; Youdim, M. Catechin polyphenols: Neurodegeneration and neuroprotection in neurodegenerative diseases. *Free Radic. Biol. Med.* **2004**, *37*, 304–317. [CrossRef] [PubMed]

29. Islam, N.; Ishita, I.; Jung, H.; Choi, J. Vicenin-2 isolated from Artemisia capillaris exhibited potent anti-glycation properties. *Food Chem. Toxicol.* **2014**, *69*, 55–62. [CrossRef] [PubMed]

30. Li, J.; Ge, R.; Tang, L.; Li, Q. Protective effects of farrerol against hydrogen-peroxide-induced apoptosis in human endothelium-derived EA.hy926 cells. *Can. J. Physiol. Pharmacol.* **2013**, *91*, 733–740. [CrossRef] [PubMed]

31. Kim, J.; Choi, S.; Cho, H.; Hwang, H.; Kim, Y.; Lim, S.; Kim, C.; Kim, H.; Peterson, S.; Shin, D. Protective effects of kaempferol (3,4',5,7-tetrahydroxyflavone) against amyloid beta peptide (Abeta)-induced neurotoxicity in ICR mice. *Biosci. Biotechnol. Biochem.* **2010**, *74*, 397–401. [CrossRef] [PubMed]

32. Tang, J.; Li, J.; Qi, W.; Qiu, W.; Li, P.; Li, B.; Song, B. Inhibition of SREBP by a small molecule, betulin, improves hyperlipidemia and insulin resistance and reduces atherosclerotic plaques. *Cell Metab.* **2011**, *13*, 44–56. [CrossRef] [PubMed]

33. Lucetti, D.; Lucetti, E.; Bandeira, M.; Veras, H.; Silva, A.; Leal, L.; Lopes, A.; Alves, V.; Silva, G.; Brito, G.; et al. Anti-inflammatory effects and possible mechanism of action of lupeol acetate isolated from Himatanthus drasticus (Mart) Plumel. *J. Inflamm.* **2010**, *7*, 60. [CrossRef] [PubMed]

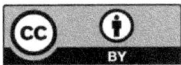

medicines

Discussion

A Reassessment of the *Marrubium Vulgare* L. Herb's Potential Role in Diabetes Mellitus Type 2: First Results Guide the Investigation toward New Horizons

Javier Rodríguez Villanueva [1,*] , Jorge Martín Esteban [2] and Laura Rodríguez Villanueva [3]

[1]   Biomedical Sciences Department, Pharmacy and Pharmaceutical Technology Unit, Faculty of Pharmacy, University of Alcalá, Ctra. de Madrid-Barcelona (Autovía A2) Km. 33,600, 28805 Alcalá de Henares, Madrid, Spain

[2]   Phytotherapy Faculty, University of Barcelona, Gran Via de les Corts Catalanes, 585, 08007 Barcelona, Spain; jorgemartinesteban@gmail.com

[3]   Faculty of Pharmacy, University of Alcalá, Ctra. de Madrid-Barcelona (Autovía A2) Km. 33,600 28805 Alcalá de Henares, Madrid, Spain; lau95.rv@gmail.com

*   Correspondence: therealworldvsme@hotmail.com; Tel.: +34-91-347-41-58

Received: 12 July 2017; Accepted: 1 August 2017; Published: 2 August 2017

Abstract: Despite the wide variety of pharmacological activities described for the *Marrubium vulgare* L. herb, amazingly, only one clinical trial can be found in scientific literature. It was designed for the evaluation of its antidiabetic activity. Worse, the outcomes of this trial were contradictory to what previous in vivo mice assays had concluded. Therefore, should *Marrubium vulgare* be ruled out due to its lack of therapeutic potential in diabetes? The authors suggest a reevaluation of the clinical trial methodology to establish valid and final results.

Keywords: *Marrubium vulgare* L. herb; diabetes mellitus type 2; clinical trial; methodology

1. Introduction

Marrubium L. (Lamiaceae) has about forty species, generally distributed in temperate regions of Central and Western Asia, North Africa, Europe, and South America. Generally, these plants are large annual or perennial shrubs [1]. The furane labdane diterpene marrubiin is assumed to be the chemotaxonomic marker among the various species of the *Marrubium* genus. Generally, marrubiin is isolated from dried whole plants of *Marrubium vulgare* Linn (white/common horehound, hoarhound, marriout, maromba, marroio-branco, or marrubio) in a proportion of 0.3–0.7% [2]. *M. vulgare* L., commonly known as "white horehound" can be identified as a robust perennial herb, with densely cottony stems and white flowers [3].

Researchers have tried to support the biological activities described for the *M. vulgare* L. herb (for an extended analysis, see Reference [4] and Figure 1) by the isolation and identification of biologically active phytochemicals such as diterpenes (marrubiin and related compounds), flavonoids (luteolin, apigenin, ladanein, quercetin, isoquercitrin, chrysoeriol, or vitexin), phenylpropanoid esters (including acteoside (or verbascoside), forsythoside B, arenarioside, ballotetroside, alyssonoide, marruboside, and acethyl marruboside), tannins (such as proanthocyanidins, catechin and epicatechin, condensed tannins), and sterols [5].

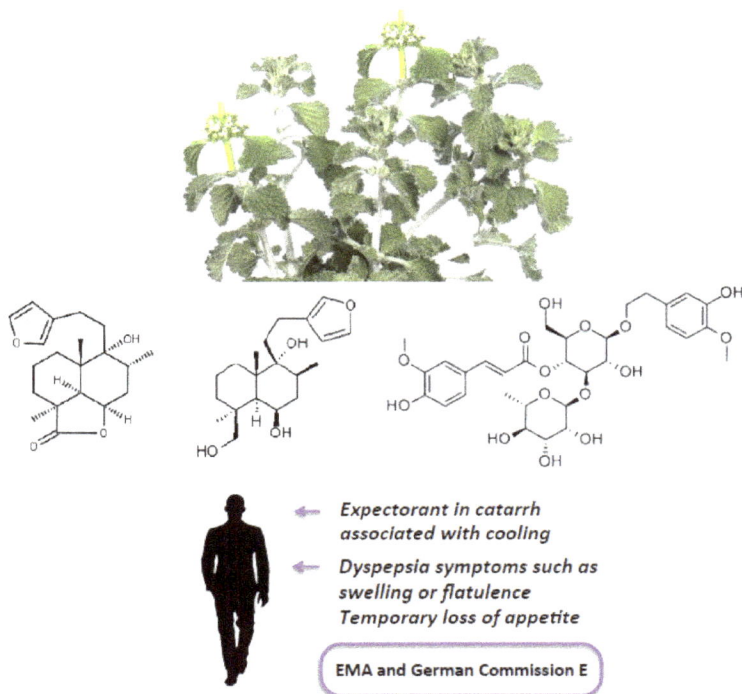

Figure 1. Top, photograph of the aerial part of *Marrubium vulgare* L.; Middle, marrubiin, marrubiol (both diterpenes), and martinoside (a phenylpropanoid), three of the plant's active compounds; Bottom, the European Medicine Agency (EMA) and German Commission E approved indications for the aerial part of *Marrubium vulgare* L.

Diabetes mellitus is a metabolic disease characterized by chronic hyperglycemia resulting from defects in insulin secretion, insulin action, or both. Diabetes mellitus type 2 (DM2), known as adult type or non-insulin-dependent diabetes mellitus, is treated by controlling the diet and oral hypoglycemic drugs [6]. In 2004, more than 120 million people in the world had diabetes. In 2015, there were approximately 415 million people with diabetes, and this is projected to increase to 642 million by 2040 (International Diabetes Federation atlas, 2015). In Mexico, DM2 affects 8.2% of the population between 20 and 69 years old and has the highest mortality rate of chronic degenerative diseases, representing 16.7% of deaths [7].

*M. Vulgar*e L. has been reported to be used in the treatment of diabetes in traditional medicine in Mexico [8] and central Morocco [6], and scientific studies have revealed through in vivo research the hypoglycemic effect of this plant, supporting its traditional use in diabetes mellitus control [9].

2. Preclinical In Vivo Observations: The Starting Point

Initial studies showed that horehound infusion (132 g of the dried plant/1 L water, in a dose of 4 mL/kg body weight) decreased the glucose curve significantly when a 50% dextrose solution (4 mL/kg of weight) was administered [10].

Years later, the methanolic extract of the top parts of *M. vulgare* L. was also evaluated for the same purpose [11], and 500 g of the aerial part was homogenized with methanol for 15 min, three times each with 1000 mL (500 g/1 × 3 L), followed by distillation of the solvent under reduced pressure. The percentage yield was calculated as 12%. In this case, diabetes was induced in rats through streptozotocin (in 0.1 M sodium citrate buffer, pH 4.5) injected intraperitoneally at a dose of 55 mg/kg, as a single dose. The diabetic rats orally received the extract of *M. vulgare* in a dose of 500 mg dry extract/kg of weight in a 1% CMC-Na vehicle once a day, starting on the 11th day. The oral administration of the *M. vulgare* extract significantly reduced the plasma glucose level after three days by more than 7% (curiously, glibenclamide has no effect here). After 14 days, the reduction was marked, reaching 42% compared to the control values of the diabetic group. The plasma glucose level was reduced in the glibenclamide group by 31% compared to the control values of the diabetic group on the 28th day.

In 2012, Boudjelal et al. [9] proved through preclinical in vivo trials the hypoglycemic and hypolipidemic effects in diabetic albino rats (180–200 g) fed ad libitum with a pellet diet and water, kept and maintained under laboratory conditions of temperature and light (24 ± 1 °C and a 12 h light/dark cycle). Rats were randomly divided into six groups and injected intraperitoneally with a single injection of alloxan monohydrate (150 mg/kg) to cause hyperglycemia and fasting blood glucose levels greater than 300 mg/dL.

The extract of *M. Vulgare* administered was prepared by boiling 6 g of the aerial parts of the plant, dried at room temperature in the dark and ground to a powder, in 25 mL of distilled water for 15 min, the mixture of which was then left to reach room temperature and filtrated. Extracts in a dose of 100, 200, or 300 mg/kg of body weight were orally administered twice daily for 15 days. The positive control was glibenclamide (5 mg/kg of body weight); a normal control and a diabetic control were also included. A sharp decline in blood glucose levels was observed from the third day after the treatment with three doses of *M. vulgare* extracts and glibenclamide (more than 5% for 300 mg/kg of body weight, and up to 12% for glibenclamide). In particular, the highest percentage decrease of glycaemia levels was observed after 28 days for the treatments with 300 mg/kg of body weight of *Marrubium* infusion (−62.55%) and the positive control glibenclamide (−65.90%). Serum glucose, total lipids, triglycerides, and total cholesterol decreased after the administration of *M. vulgare* extract in all doses without attaining the values of the normal control. The effect was similar to that observed with the positive control, glibenclamide. The authors attribute these results to a stimulation of insulin secretion from beta cells of islets and/or inhibition of insulin degradation processes due to the high content of flavonoids in the drug (15.53 mg quercetin equivalent/g of dry plant material).

In both studies, there were no physical signs of toxicity, such as writhing, gasping, palpitation and respiratory rate, or mortality in the rats. The rats treated with different doses of *M. vulgare* did not show any drug-induced behavioral disorders.

3. From Animals to Humans: The Clinical Trial Issue for Herbal Medicine

More than 10 years ago, Wolsko and coworkers [12] stated that poor quality control in the United States was not surprising, given the US regulatory environment as dictated by the Dietary Supplement Health and Education Act of 1994. The same could be applied nowadays, for the United States as well as for the European Union. There is still currently no minimum standard of practice for manufacturing dietary supplements, no premarket safety or efficacy studies are needed, and dietary supplements do not need approval from the Food and Drug Administration (FDA) or the European Medicine Agency (EMA) before they are marketed. It continues to be purely the manufacturers' responsibility to ensure that supplements are safe and labeled properly before marketing. The FDA or the EMA (coordinated with the agency of each member state) can take action to restrict a product's use only after it has been shown that a dietary supplement is unsafe, sometimes years later, when it has taken the lives or has cost the health of innocent people. In the absence of evidence to the contrary, herbal supplements used in clinical trials have the same poor quality as demonstrated in the marketplace as a whole. This fact, linked with the number of pharmacognosy drugs of the same species and the different treatments being undergone, makes it very difficult if not impossible to establish valid conclusions that are not contradictory to what has been reported before in animals.

For the *Marrubium vulgare* L. herb, while some articles describe and sustain the ethnopharmacological use [13], only one clinical trial can be found in the scientific literature up to date [7]. This is striking given that, in 2015, preparations of this species were the best-selling herbal dietary supplements, reaching approximately $106 million in retail sales [14]. This randomized, double-blind, and controlled clinical trial was conducted to evaluate the clinical effect produced by its aqueous extract on type 2 non-controlled diabetes mellitus. The verum product consisted of fresh *M. vulgare* L. leaves that were dried under environmental temperatures and protected from direct light and then milled. Ethylene oxide was used for sterilization. Patients had to prepare the treatment immediately before administration. A 1-g filter-paper envelope was placed in a cup of boiling water for 5 min. *M. vulgare* L. extract was administered three times a day, before every meal. The infusion was analyzed through HPLC with UV detection at 255 nm only for chlorogenic acid determination. This compound was not found in the extract.

Outpatients of either sex, between 30 and 60 years old, who had been diagnosed with type 2 diabetes no more than five years earlier, were selected. All patients were under medical treatment but showing a fasting blood glucose >140 mg/dL. As usual, patients affected with diabetes complications or nephropathy, pregnant women, patients with gestational diabetes, and hospitalized patients were not selected. In this study, insulin-dependent or type I diabetics were excluded, and, for comfort and to assure results, people who needed to travel frequently were also not selected. A total of 43 patients were recruited, and 21 received an *M. vulgare* L. infusion. The other 22 received a *Cecropia obtusifolia* extract. All patients showed treatment adherence, evaluated by counting the used dosages.

The study was carried out for 21 days. Prior to infusion administration, every seven days and after the clinical trial, the fasting determination of glucose, cholesterol, triglycerides, urea, creatinine, and uric acid in blood was carried out using automatic equipment (Autolab) with standardized techniques by a certified external laboratory.

In this study, effectiveness was considered a decrease in the basal concentration of glucose, cholesterol, or triglycerides by at least 25%. *M. vulgare* L. caused that effect in only two of the 21 patients (9.52%). The mean of plasma glucose level was reduced by 0.64%, and that of cholesterol and triglycerides by 4.16% and 5.78%, respectively. These results were disappointing.

4. Some Result Considerations Must Be Kept in Mind: Paving the Way for Future Actions

Nevertheless, some considerations must be taken into account. First of all, as the authors state, a crude extract was evaluated, with a similar preparation to that used in traditional medicine. As previously described, effective results on animal models were obtained after the administration of specific extracts, available after processing crude plant material with different methods. The effect of preparation methods on composition or content (as well as on undesired ingredients) is not fully understood. The same applies for therapeutic activity. Also, the administration route influences the bioavailability, pharmacological activity, and clinical effectiveness of a phytotherapeutic preparation. Previously, clinical studies could only demonstrate observations if the botanic drug material and the study design were rationally based on that basis.

What is important here is that 6-octadecynoic acid, a fatty acid with a triple bond found in *Marrubium vulgare* L., exhibits PPARγ agonist activity by directly binding to helix 12 through the conformational change of the Ω loop. Compounds with PPARγ agonist activity have been clinically used for treatment of type 2 diabetes by improving insulin resistance [15]. However, it is only found in the organic (methanolic) extract of the aerial parts (tops, leaves, and flowers), as fatty acids are not soluble in water infusion. It is not difficult to propose that, between others, there may be a presumable relation between the efficacy of the methanolic extract in mice models/lack of efficacy as an aqueous extraction and the presence/absence of 6-octadecynoic acid.

Despite this, as we previously stated [16], a characterized compound with a perfectly defined mechanism of action at a particular dose fulfills the negative requirements (such as toxicity) inherited from classical pharmacology. However, new trends suggest an integrative approach in which a wide variety of compounds act on multiple targets together to produce a final action through a balance resulting from minor changes (synergy); something different is not expected here. Diterpenes, flavonoids, and phenylpropanoid esters may also play a role in the antidiabetic activity or in the diabetes concomitant effects as on animal models.

No less important is a diligent analysis of the dose translation from animals to humans, if possible with recognized recommendations (i.e., FDA, EMA, or Commission E if available). Elberry and colleagues [11] administered to rats 500 mg of dried extract (as previously described) per kg of weight. For an average person (weighing 60 kg), this dosage correlates with a dose of 81 mg/kg of weight. Taking into account the drug/extraction ratio, almost 39 g of the herbal substance (crude drug) is needed, which is impossible to achieve for an individual administration (the EMA recommends a 1–2 g dose of the cut drug, and the German Commission E recommends a 4–5 g dose of the fresh/dried plant material per day). Considering the hypothesis that 6-octadecynoic acid is the compound primarily involved in the antidiabetic activity and available in sufficient amounts of raw material, these results reveal that a more efficient extraction method should be developed (ethyl acetate showed good results in the study by Ohtera et al. [15], but possible toxicity risks must be abolished before achieving clinical trials with EtOAc extracts).

For example, we proposed that the extract prepared by El Bardai et al. [17,18] was obtained by aqueous infusion (5 g air parts/100 mL of water, yield after lyophilization) with a drug: extract ratio (DER) 6.2:1 and performance 13%. This extract minimizes possible toxicity due to organic solvents, allows oral administration, and makes feasible the fulfilment of the recommended therapeutic range, which allows a maximum amount of 6 g per drug per day.

Finally, it is important to notice the slighter side effects (described by one in every four patients) in the clinical trial, including nausea, oral dryness, sialorrhea, dizziness, and anorexia, although they were not adverse enough to necessarily cause a withdrawal from the study [7]. These results and the acquired experience in the traditional intake of the water infusion of *Marrubium vulgare* L. can be considered safe. In spite of this, the number of patients, as is usual in clinical trials of herb preparations, was reduced, and the establishment of general conclusions is therefore almost impossible.

Conflicts of Interest: The authors declare that there is no conflict of interest.

References

1. Kahkeshani, N.; Gharedaghi, M.; Hadjiakhoondi, A.; Sharifzadeh, M. Antinociceptive effect of extracts of Marrubium astracanicum Jacq. aerial parts. *Avicenna J. Phytomed.* **2017**, *7*, 73–79. [PubMed]
2. Mittal, V.; Nanda, A. Intensification of marrubiin concentration by optimization of microwave-assisted (low CO_2 yielding) extraction process for *Marrubium vulgare* using central composite design and antioxidant evaluation. *Pharm. Biol.* **2017**, *55*, 1337–1347. [CrossRef] [PubMed]
3. Aouni, R.; Attia, M.B.; Jaafoura, M.H.; Bibi-Derbel, A. Effects of the hydro-ethanolic extract of *Marrubium vulgare* in female rats. *Asian Pac. J. Trop. Med.* **2017**, *10*, 160–164. [CrossRef] [PubMed]
4. Villanueva, R.J.; Esteban, M.J. An Insight into a Blockbuster Phytomedicine; *Marrubium vulgare* L. Herb. More of a Myth than a Reality? *Phytother. Res.* **2016**, *30*, 1551–1558. [CrossRef] [PubMed]
5. Garjani, A.; Tila, D.; Hamedeyazdan, S.; Vaez, H. An investigation on cardioprotective potential of *Marrubium vulgare* aqueous fraction against ischemia-reperfusion injury in isolated rat heart. *Folia Morphol. (Warsz)* **2015**. [CrossRef] [PubMed]
6. Barkaoui, M.; Katiri, A.; Boubaker, H.; Msanda, F. Ethnobotanical survey of medicinal plants used in the traditional treatment of diabetes in Chtouka Ait Baha and Tiznit (Western Anti-Atlas), Morocco. *J. Ethnopharmacol.* **2017**, *198*, 338–350. [CrossRef] [PubMed]
7. Herrera-Arellano, A.; Aguilar-Santamaria, L.; Garcia-Hernandez, B.; Nicasio-Torres, P. Clinical trial of Cecropia obtusifolia and *Marrubium vulgare* leaf extracts on blood glucose and serum lipids in type 2 diabetics. *Phytomedicine* **2004**, *11*, 561–566. [CrossRef] [PubMed]

8. Argueta, V.A.; Cano, L.M.; Rodarte, M.E. (Eds.) *Atlas de las Plantas de la Medicina Tradicional Mexicana*; Instituto Nacional Indigenista: Mexico DF, República de Mexico, 1994; Volume 3. Available online: www.medicinatradicionalmexicana.unam.mx/monografia.php?=3&t=Marrubio&id=7620l (accessed on 29 July 2017).

9. Boudjelal, A.; Henchiri, C.; Siracusa, L.; Sari, M. Compositional analysis and in vivo anti-diabetic activity of wild Algerian *Marrubium vulgare* L. infusion. *Fitoterapia* **2012**, *83*, 286–292. [CrossRef] [PubMed]

10. Roman Ramos, R.; Alarcon-Aguilar, F.; Lara-Lemus, A.; Flores-Saenz, J.L. Hypoglycemic effect of plants used in Mexico as antidiabetics. *Arch. Med. Res.* **1992**, *23*, 59–64. [PubMed]

11. Elberry, A.A.; Harraz, F.M.; Ghareib, S.A.; Gabr, S.A. Methanolic extract of *Marrubium vulgare* ameliorates hyperglycemia and dyslipidemia in streptozotocin-induced diabetic rats. *Int. J. Diabetes Mellit.* **2015**, *3*, 37–44. [CrossRef]

12. Wolsko, P.M.; Solondz, D.K.; Phillips, R.S.; Schachter, S.C. Lack of herbal supplement characterization in published randomized controlled trials. *Am. J. Med.* **2005**, *118*, 1087–1093. [CrossRef] [PubMed]

13. Ballero, M.; Sotgiu, A.M.; Piu, G. Empirical administration of preparations of *Marrubium vulgare* in the asthmatic syndrome. *Biomed. Lett.* **1998**, *57*, 31–36.

14. Izzo, A.A.; Hoon-Kim, S.; Radhakrishnan, R.; Williamson, E.M. A Critical Approach to Evaluating Clinical Efficacy, Adverse Events and Drug Interactions of Herbal Remedies. *Phytother. Res.* **2016**, *30*, 691–700. [CrossRef] [PubMed]

15. Ohtera, A.; Miyamae, Y.; Nakai, N.; Kawachi, A. Identification of 6-octadecynoic acid from a methanol extract of *Marrubium vulgare* L. as a peroxisome proliferator-activated receptor gamma agonist. *Biochem. Biophys. Res. Commun.* **2013**, *440*, 204–209. [CrossRef] [PubMed]

16. Villanueva, J.R.; Esteban, J.M.; Villanueva, R.L. Solving the puzzle: What is behind our forefathers' anti-inflammatory remedies? *J. Int. Ethnopharmacol.* **2017**, *6*, 128–143. [CrossRef] [PubMed]

17. El Bardai, S.; Hamaide, M.C.; Lyoussi, B.; Quetin-Leclercq, J.; Morel, N.; Wibo, M. Marrubenol interacts with the phenylalkylamine binding site of the L-type calcium channel. *Eur. J. Pharmacol.* **2004**, *492*, 269–272. [CrossRef] [PubMed]

18. El Bardai, S.; Lyoussi, B.; Wibo, M.; Morel, N. Comparative study of the antihypertensive activity of *Marrubium vulgare* and of the dihydropyridine calciumantagonistamlodipine in spontaneously hypertensive rat. *Clin. Exp. Hypertens.* **2004**, *26*, 465–474. [CrossRef] [PubMed]

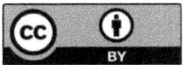

medicines

MDPI

Case Report

Successful Pregnancy after Treatment with Chinese Herbal Medicine in a 43-Year-Old Woman with Diminished Ovarian Reserve and Multiple Uterus Fibrosis: A Case Report

Benqi Teng [1,2], Jie Peng [1,3], Madeleine Ong [1] and Xianqin Qu [1,*]

1   School of Life Sciences, University of Technology Sydney, NSW 2007, Australia;
    tengbq@mail.sysu.edu.cn (B.T.); PengJie528@outlook.com (J.P.); Madeleine.L.Ong@student.uts.edu.au (M.O.)
2   Department of Obstetrics, The Third Affiliated Hospital of Sun Yat-sen University, 600 Tianhe Road,
    Guangzhou 510630, China
3   Department of Gynaecology and Obstetrics, Suzhou Wuzhong People's Hospital, Suzhou 215128, China
*   Correspondence: Xianqin.Qu@uts.edu.au; Tel.: +61-2-9514-7852; Fax: +61-2-9514-8206

Academic Editor: James D. Adams
Received: 15 December 2016; Accepted: 4 February 2017; Published: 9 February 2017

Abstract: Objective: To highlight a natural approach to coexisting oligomenorrhea, subfertility, luteal phase insufficiency and multiple fibroids cohesively when in vitro fertilisation (IVF) has failed. **Case Presentation:** A 43-year-old woman with diminished ovarian reserve and multiple uterine fibroids had previously been advised to discontinue IVF treatment. According to Chinese Medicine diagnosis, herbal formulae were prescribed for improving age-related ovarian insufficiency as well as to control the growth of fibroids. After 4 months of treatment, the patient's menstrual cycle became regular and plasma progesterone one week after ovulation increased from 10.9 nmol/L to 44.9 nmol/L. After 6 months, she achieved a natural conception, resulting in a live birth of a healthy infant at an estimated gestational age of 40 weeks. **Conclusions:** The successful treatment with Chinese Herbal Medicine for this case highlights a natural therapy to manage infertility due to ovarian insufficiency and multiple fibroids after unsuccessful IVF outcome.

Keywords: Chinese herbal medicine; diminished ovarian reserve; infertility; in vitro fertilization; uterus fibrosis

1. Introduction

Advanced maternal age contributes to subfertility due to diminished ovarian reserve (DOR) and decreased oocyte quality [1]. Reduced fertility potential may also be attributable to uterine fibroids which are more prevalent in women aged over 30 [2] depending on their size and location, which can affect embryo implantation [3]. Indeed, women with DOR and fibroids have a significantly low fertility rate despite advanced in vitro fertilization (IVF) techniques [4]. Given the limited treatment options after failure in IVF with DOR, these women often seek alternative therapy, such as Traditional Chinese medicine (TCM) to reserve adoption or using donor's egg as the last option.

Chinese medicinal herbs have been used for more than two thousand years to treat gynaecological disorders including infertility. In the last decades, experimental and clinical studies have shown that these herbal ingredients can regulate gonadotropin-releasing hormone and ovarian sex hormone levels to induce ovulation and promote blood flow to the ovaries to improve ovarian reserve [5]. TCM is unique as it applies a formula with multiple natural ingredients that are capable of counteracting complex endocrine and reproductive disorders. Here, we present a successful live birth with Chinese herbal medicine (CHM) treatment to a 43-year-old nulliparous woman with DOR and uterus fibroids after failed conception from IVF.

2. Case Presentation

A 43-year-old woman visited our clinic for CHM treatment of infertility. She reached menarche at 13 years of age and at this time her menstrual cycle was regular with a normal menstrual flow. Oral contraceptive pills were taken from age 21–23 and she had no previous pregnancies prior to our treatment. She started trying to conceive at age 40 and her husband, aged 41, had no remarkable health problems and normal semen analysis as defined by the World Health Organization 2010 criteria [6]. After two years of trying to achieve natural conception, she was referred to a fertility specialist for IVF treatment. Prior to the initiation of treatment, a pelvic ultrasound showed that the right ovary was not visible and the left ovary measured 2.7 mL with only 3 antral follicles and both fallopian tubes were clearly patent. The uterus was bulky measuring at $103 \times 125 \times 68$ mm with multiple fibroids including two larger subserosal fibroids. Serum anti-mullerian hormone (AMH) level of <3 pmol/L was within the <25% percentile for correlated age. Hormone testing on day 5 of her menstrual cycle identified follicle stimulating hormone (FSH) levels of 1.9 IU/L (normal range 1.5–10), luteinising hormone (LH) levels of 2.8 IU/L (normal range 2.0–12), Oestradiol (E2) levels of 913 pmol/L (normal range <320) and Progesterone (P) levels of <0.5 nmol/L (normal range 0.3–4.0). According to the ESHRE criteria this patient had suspected poor ovarian response [7]. Therefore, controlled ovarian hyperstimulation (COH) with daily FSH injections from day 3 of her cycle was applied for oocyte retrieval, however, only one mature oocyte was collected, and she failed to conceive after fertilized embryo transferring. The fertility specialist therefore advised her to seek egg donation or cease IVF. The patient consequently sought out treatment at our Chinese Medicine clinic in hope of achieving fertility.

At the time the patient visited the clinic her menstrual cycles ranged between 24 and 42 days. According to the diagnosis, basic formula containing 10 herbs was prescribed (Table 1), aiming to (1) improve diminished ovarian function and regulate the menstrual cycle and (2) restrain the growth of uterus fibroids which corresponds to tonifying vital essence and regulating and nourishing blood in TCM.

Table 1. Description of Chinese Herbal Formula and Possible Pharmacological Effects [8,9].

Herb Name	TCM Action	Possible Pharmacological Effects
Shu Di Huang (Radix *Rehmannia glutinosa*)	Tonifies Qi and Blood.	Improves blood supply to reproductive tissue.
Dang Gui (Radix *Angelicae sinensis*)	Tonifies and moves blood.	Improves blood supply to reproductive tissue and organs. Improves ovarian function.
Tu Si Zi (Semen *Cuscutae chinensis*)	Consolidates vital essence.	Promotes fertility by improving the quality of oocyte.
Sang Shen Zi (*Fructus mori*)	Strengthens vital essence.	Anti-oxidant and improves the quality of the oocyte. Anti-ageing properties.
Gou Qi Zi (*Fructus lycii*)	Nourishes blood.	Scavenges free radicals, increases DNA synthesis in reproductive tissue.
Ba Ji Tian (Radix *Morindae officinalis*)	Supports the vital essence.	Stimulates pituitary gland to improve ovulation.
Dan Shen (Radix *Salvia miltiorrhizae*)	Dissolves blood stasis.	Anti-inflammatory, promotes microcirculation to reproductive organs.
Bai Shao (Radix *Paeoniae lactiflorae*)	Nourish blood, regulate qi.	Anti-inflammatory.
Xia Ku Cao (Spica *Prunellae vulgaris*)	Dissolves mass formation.	Anti-fibrotic.
E Zhu (Rhizoma *Curcuma phaeocaulis*)	Dissolves blood stasis.	Anti-fibrotic.

Abbreviations: TCM: Traditional Chinese Medicine. Possible pharmacological effects were derived from.

The herbal mixture was decocted into 500 mL and divided into two drinks daily. Ovulation was monitored by basal body temperature (BBT) and ovulation prediction kit. Plasma progesterone was measured one week of ovulation revealed by BBT chart and LH surge. Following initial consult and first month treatment with CHM, the patient underwent hormone testing one week after ovulation: P was 10.9 nmol/L, LH was 0.8 IU/L (normal range 2.0–12), FSH was 2.0 IU/L (normal range 1.5–10), E2 was 184 pmol/L (normal range 125–1300). After 12 weeks of treatment, the patient's menstrual cycle became regular with cycle lengthen between 30 and 35 days. Pelvic ultrasound on day 9 of cycle indicated ovaries of both sides were normal in size and uterine size was reduced with measuring 84 × 62 × 56 mm as well as decreased sizes of intramural and subserosal fibroids. A blood test was also performed at day 23 of her menstrual cycle (about one week after ovulation) and revealed improvement of progesterone levels from 10.9 up to 28.1 nmol/L.

From week 13, the formula was slightly modified according to the follicular phase by adding Radix *Polygoni multiflori* (*He Shou Wu*) 10 g to nourish blood, and in the luteal phase by adding Radix Dipsaci (*Xu Duan*) 12 g and Cortex *Eucommiae ulmoidis* (*Du Zhong*) 9 g to assist in embryo implantation. Anti-fibrosis herb, *Prunellae vulgaris* and Rhizoma *Curcuma phaeocaulis* had been ceased after 4 months of treatment. After 5 months of taking CHM, although AMH was at 1.3 pmol/L, plasma progesterone levels after one week of ovulation went from 10.9 nmol/L to 44.9 nmol/L, suggesting that the quality of oocyte and function of corpus luteum had been improved. After 6 months of treatment with CHM, she achieved natural conception, resulting in a live birth of a healthy female infant weighing 3350 g at an estimated gestational age of 40 weeks through caesarean section. No modifications to the lifestyle of the patient were made during this period.

3. Discussion

The conventional approaches to sterility include ovulation induction, intrauterine insemination and IVF. In this case, woman with advanced maternal age, IVF may be the most successful technique to achieve conception. However, because of the DOR, this patient presented a very poor response to COH, resulting in unsuccessful IVF. Consequently, the patient turned to CHM. Our treatment achieved pregnancy and a healthy live birth with Chinese herbal formulae containing herbs supporting the folliculogenesis cycle, invigorating blood, improving microcirculation, and resolving masses to benefit both ovary and uterus.

Chinese herbal medicines have long been used for the treatment of infertility. Numerous studies demonstrated that CHM could regulate the gonadotropin-releasing hormone (GnRH) to induce ovulation and improve the uterus blood flow and menstrual changes of endometrium [10,11]. An advantage of CHM treatment is that it utilizes individualized formulas tailored to a patient's condition. In this case, non-invasive treatment with CHM targeted two major causes underlying her infertility simultaneously, including poor quality of oocyte due to diminished ovarian reserve and uterine fibroids. The successful pregnancy eventually achieved through improvement of uterus environment and enhanced ovarian function.

It is generally accepted that submucosal fibroids but not subserosal fibroids have a negative impact on fertility by the virtue of their involvement in the endometrial cavity. This patient had multiple large subserosal and intramural fibroids of equal proportions. It has also been confirmed that myomas have higher levels of aromatase converting estrogens to estradiol, resulting in an imbalance of estradiol and progesterone, which is detrimental to embryo implantation and contributes to miscarriage [3]. In this infertility case, uterine fibroids have been considered as a treatment target because the estradiol levels of 913 pmol/L (normal range <320) was significantly high at follicular phase and there was also evidence of a bulky uterus caused by multiple fibroids. The large subserosal and intramural fibroids affect the endometrium homogeneous and may have negative impact on the embryo implantation on her natural conception and during IVF procedure. It is also a concern that these fibroids may aggressively grow during the pregnancy because of the ovarian hormone surge, subsequently affecting foetus development.

The herbal formula used in this case is able to balance *yin* and *yang*, nourish blood and invigorate blood circulation from a TCM perspective. In medical science, the CHM formula may restore ovarian function through improving blood flow to reproductive organs, regulating hormone secretions, lowering systemic inflammation as well as having anti-tumour properties. Among of them, Radix *Salvia miltiorrhizae*, Radix *Paeoniae lactiflorae*, Spica *Prunellae vulgaris* and Rhizoma *Curcuma phaeocaulis* have strong effects on blood stasis which is involved in mass (fibroids) formation in the reproductive system. Pharmacological studies have shown that these herbs reduce inflammation and inhibit neoplasia [12,13]. Meanwhile, the combination of Radix *Rehmannia glutinosa*, Semen *Cuscutae chinensis*, *Fructus mori*, *Fructus lycii*, Radix *Morindae officinalis* are commonly used in infertility due to ovarian factors, such as PCOS and primary ovarian insufficiency [13–16]. However, the precise mechanisms of Chinese herbs remain unclear with further research warranted.

After one month of treatment, day 6 oestradiol levels of 930 pmol/L reduced to 387 pmol/L. At the month five of the treatment, plasma progesterone from 10.9 nmol/L raised to 44.9 nmol/L, indicating improved ovarian function. Meanwhile, the size of the fibroids had shrunk with an overall reduced size of the uterus. These results indicate that CHM treatment inhibited fibroid growth and improved ovarian function, and may suggest enhanced quality of oocyte, evidenced by regularity of menstrual cycle, mid-cycle ovulation and elevated progesterone levels at luteal phase. Evidence suggests that oocyte quality profoundly affects fertilisation and embryo development [17]. The treatment achieved this woman's natural pregnancy, suggesting the improvement of oocyte quality. The limitation in this case observation is that other assessments for oocyte quality such as morphological character of oocyte and corpus luteum and other biomarkers, such as mitochondrial status and glucose-6-phosphate dehydrogenase 1 activity and apoptosis of follicular cells, were not measured.

Infertility is a life-altering burden and the disorder affects a couple's emotional health and wellness. Given the limited treatment options after failure in IVF, women with DOR who intend to get pregnant have to rely on assisted reproductive technology using donor eggs. The procedure is costly and only has a live birth rate of ~30% [4] and contributes to psychological distress. The results of this case demonstrate that CHM is capable of targeting multiple reproductive abnormalities involved in infertility. More specifically, herbal medicine can improve ovarian function and prevent inevitable miscarriage related to luteal phase defect and multiple fibroids. The successful treatment with CHM for this case highlights the potential of a natural approach to coexisting oligomenorrhea, subfertility, luteal phase insufficiency and multiple fibroids cohesively. CHM therapy offers a hope for aged women who have failed IVF cycles and decide to pursue parenthood with their own oocytes. The repeatability of CHM on infertility should be warranted through rigorously designed clinical trials.

Acknowledgments: We are thankful to our patient for her willingness to use her anonymized data for this publication.

Conflicts of Interest: The authors declare no conflict of interest.

References

1.	Gurtcheff, S.E.; Klein, N.A. Diminished ovarian reserve and infertility. *Clin. Obstet. Gynecol.* **2011**, *54*, 666–674. [CrossRef] [PubMed]

2.	Purohit, P.; Vigneswaran, K. Fibroids and Infertility. *Curr. Obstet. Gynecol. Rep.* **2016**, *5*, 81–88. [CrossRef] [PubMed]

3.	Vitale, S.G.; Padula, F.; Gulino, F.A. Management of uterine fibroids in pregnancy: Recent trends. *Curr. Opin. Obstet. Gynecol.* **2015**, *27*, 432–437. [CrossRef] [PubMed]

4.	Nelson, L.M. Clinical practice. Primary ovarian insufficiency. *N. Engl. J. Med.* **2009**, *360*, 606–614. [CrossRef] [PubMed]

5.	Zhang, C.; Xu, X. Advancement in the treatment of diminished ovarian reserve by traditional Chinese and Western medicine. *Exp. Ther. Med.* **2016**, *11*, 1173–1176. [CrossRef] [PubMed]

6. Coope, T.G.; Noonan, E.; von Eckardstein, S.; Auger, J.; Baker, G.; Behre, H.M.; Haugen, T.B.; Kruger, T.; Wang, C.; Mbizvo, M.T.; et al. World Health Organization Reference Values for Human Semen Characteristics. *Hum. Reprod. Update* **2010**, *16*, 231–245. [CrossRef] [PubMed]

7. Ferraretti, A.P.; La Marca, A.; Fauser, B.C.; Tarlatzis, B.; Nargund, G.; Gianaroli, L.; ESHRE Working Group on Poor Ovarian Response Definition. ESHRE consensus on the definition of 'poor response' to ovarian stimulation for in vitro fertilization: The Bologna criteria. *Hum. Reprod.* **2011**, *26*, 1616–1624. [CrossRef] [PubMed]

8. Chen, J.K.; Chen, T.T. *Chinese Medical Herbology and Pharmacology*, 1st ed.; Art of Medicine Press Inc.: City of Industry, CA, USA, 2001.

9. Shen, Y.J. *Pharmacology of Chinese Herbal Medicine*, 1st ed.; People's Medical Publishing House: Beijing, China, 2000.

10. Huang, S.T.; Chen, A.P. Traditional Chinese medicine and infertility. *Curr. Opin. Obstet. Gynecol.* **2008**, *20*, 211–215. [CrossRef] [PubMed]

11. Lee, S.H.; Kwak, S.C.; Kim, D.K.; Park, S.W.; Kim, H.S.; Kim, Y.S.; Kim, Y.; Lee, D.; Lee, J.W.; Lee, C.G.; et al. Effects of Huang Bai (*Phellodendri Cortex*) and Three Other Herbs on GnRH and GH Levels in GT1–7 and GH3 Cells. *Evid. Based Complement. Alternat. Med.* **2016**, *2016*, 9389028. [CrossRef] [PubMed]

12. Chen, X.X.; Lin, W.L.; Yeung, W.F.; Song, T.H.; Lao, L.X.; Zhang, Y.B.; Meng, W. Quality and safety control of Tumor-Shrinking Decoction (TSD), a Chinese herbal preparation for the treatment of uterine fibroids. *Biotechnol. Appl. Biochem.* **2015**. [CrossRef] [PubMed]

13. Hu, Q.; Noor, M.; Wong, Y.F.; Hylands, P.J.; Simmonds, M.S.; Xu, Q.; Jiang, D.; Hendry, B.M.; Xu, Q. In vitro anti-fibrotic activities of herbal compounds and herbs. *Nephrol. Dial. Transplant.* **2009**, *24*, 3033–3041. [CrossRef] [PubMed]

14. Hung, Y.C.; Kao, C.W.; Lin, C.C.; Liao, Y.N.; Wu, B.Y.; Hung, I.L.; Hu, W.L. Chinese Herbal Products for Female Infertility in Taiwan: A Population-Based Cohort Study. *Medicine (Baltimore)* **2016**, *95*, e3075. [CrossRef] [PubMed]

15. Ong, M.; Peng, J.; Jin, X.L.; Qu, X. Chinese Herbal Medicine for the Optimal Management of Polycystic Ovary Syndrome. *Am. J. Chin.* **2017**, in press.

16. Chao, S.L.; Huang, L.W.; Yen, H.R. Pregnancy in premature ovarian failure after therapy using Chinese herbal medicine. *Chang. Gung Med. J.* **2003**, *26*, 449–452. [PubMed]

17. Wang, Q.; Sun, Q.Y. Evaluation of oocyte quality: Morphological, cellular and molecular predictors. *Reprod. Fertil. Dev.* **2007**, *19*, 1–12. [CrossRef] [PubMed]

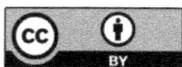

MDPI

St. Alban-Anlage 66

4052 Basel

Switzerland

Tel. +41 61 683 77 34

Fax +41 61 302 89 18

www.mdpi.com

Medicines Editorial Office

E-mail: medicines@mdpi.com

www.mdpi.com/journal/medicines

www.ingramcontent.com/pod-product-compliance
Lightning Source LLC
Chambersburg PA
CBHW051910210326
41597CB00033B/6102